The Multifidus
Back Pain Solution

Simple Exercises That Target the Muscles That Count

Jim Johnson, P.T.

Foreword by Scott D. Boden, M.D.

New Harbinger Publications, Inc.

Distributed in Canada by Raincoast Books.

Copyright © 2002 by Jim Johnson
        New Harbinger Publications, Inc.
        5674 Shattuck Avenue
        Oakland, CA 94609

Cover design © 2001 by Lightbourne
Edited by Carole Honeychurch
Text design by Tracy Marie Carlson
Drawings by Eunice Johnson

ISBN 1-57224-278-7 Paperback

New Harbinger Publications' Web site address: www.newharbinger.com

07   06   05

15   14   13   12   11   10   9   8   7

To my dad, who gave me the best piece of advice anyone's ever given me, "Make your time count for you," and my mom, who always seems to know just what to say.

One's best success comes after their
greatest disappointments.

—Henry Ward Beecher

It has been my experience that in order to be comprehensive, coherent, and concise about a particular topic, a person has to possess vast knowledge of it. Therefore, it came as no surprise to me that Jim Johnson's book, *The Multifidus Back-Pain Solution*, is thorough, logical, and brief. Jim is my physical therapist, and that is exactly the way he is when I visit him as a patient. During my therapy sessions, I have often asked Jim questions relating to my back problem, and he diligently covers every aspect of the problem, referring to "Seymour" (his office skeleton) to make sure I understand what he is referring to. In addition, he presents this information in a style that is easy to understand and remember.

Knowing how hard it is to translate from the spoken word to the written word, I found it quite an accomplishment that Jim has achieved in his book the attributes I mentioned above. In fact, while reading the manuscript, it was as if Jim was actually speaking directly to me.

Jim points out that there may be complicated physical and psychological origins of back pain. However, a significant portion of such problems is related to the functioning of the multifidus muscle. It is therefore a strong point of this book that the lay person will find the technical characteristics of the relationship between the multifidus muscle and back pain are easy to understand. In addition, this explanation of the multifidus muscle prepares the reader to understand the justification for the exercises he recommends. I have started on this exercise regimen myself and can attest to its benefits.

I have over the years come across articles, books, TV programs, and the like that claim to have a cure for some physical or psychological problem. I have found a simple rule of thumb that usually separates the serious from the opportunistic authors: the extent to which their claims are supported by reliable and valid research. The reader will find that Jim has supported all of his suggestions for curing back pain with reliable and valid research evidence.

Although the back-pain sufferer will find that the chapter titled "Information *Every* Back-Pain Sufferer Needs to Know" is worth the price of the book, they will, most importantly, find that the relief they may find by following Jim's suggestions to reduce their back pain is priceless.

—Norman Markel, Ph.D.
Atlanta, Georgia
October 17, 2001

Contents

Acknowledgments

I would like to thank everybody at New Harbinger who was involved in one way or another, be it big or small, in the publishing of this book. There is much more involved in the making of a book than simply putting ideas on paper, and it is indeed a group effort. In particular, I would like to thank Pat Fanning for his support and giving this book an opportunity to be published, and Carole Honeychurch for bringing such clarity to my writing.

Above all, to my wife, Cathy, the person single-handedly responsible for me becoming a physical therapist, which has enabled me to help so many people. She has truly made me a better person.

Foreword

Four out of every five people will experience low-back pain at some time during their life. Fortunately, most will improve with little or no treatment. Unfortunately, a limited number may develop intermittent, recurrent, or chronic symptoms. Low-back pain is the most common cause of disability in older working Americans. By selecting this book you have wisely chosen to gain an increased understanding of one of our greatest public health problems.

The Multifidus Back-Pain Solution was written specifically for you, the back-pain sufferer. It uses simple terms and clearly explains many of the most important basic concepts about your back, its health, and its potential problems. Moreover, rather than offering one author's personal opinion or beliefs, it is largely based on studies (evidence) from scientific medical journals.

Another strength of this book lies in the fact that the author is a physical therapist. One of the safest and most commonly prescribed treatments for low-back pain is exercise and/or physical therapy of some kind. Thus, the author has spent his career listening and talking to patients like you.

In summary, reading this book will help you understand your back and be better equipped to comprehend information and decisions presented to you by your health-care professionals. In addition, the detailed exercise program will make it easy for you to begin to take control of your back and make positive changes in your life. I am certain you will find this book worthwhile!

    —Scott D. Boden, M.D.
     Professor of Orthopaedic Surgery, Director,
     The Emory Spine Center Clinical Director,
     The Whitesides Orthopaedic Research Laboratory
     Emory University School of Medicine

Introduction

The best way to escape from your problem is to solve it.

—Robert Anthony

My name is Jim Johnson and I'm a physical therapist with a special interest in your particular problem—low-back pain. I've been in the trenches treating back-pain patients such as yourself for over a decade now, and I'd like to welcome you to what I hope will be one of the most helpful books on back pain that you will ever read. What will make this one of the most helpful books, you ask? Let me give you a few quick reasons why I say this:

- This book is entirely evidenced based. Sitting on the shelves behind my desk at the hospital where I work are literally hundreds of articles from peer-reviewed journals I have read over the years. I organized these articles by subject in black binders and pulled all the information for this book from them. Where I do offer my opinion in the book, I directly state it. *This book is not based upon intuition, single case reports, opinions of authorities, anecdotal evidence, or unsystematic clinical observations—unlike some books on back pain and its treatment.*

◉ I will explain in simple terms the kind of problems that many people with low-back pain can have with a little-known muscle in your back called the *multifidus*. As you will find out, cases of multifidus dysfunction have been identified and published in many peer-reviewed journals in the medical field.

◉ I will illustrate and discuss how the research has demonstrated that various traditional low-back pain diagnoses, some that you may have been labeled with, such as a "slipped disk" or chronic low-back pain, can go hand in hand with multifidus muscle problems.

◉ By reading this book you will learn a step-by-step program showing you *exactly* how to go about strengthening your multifidus muscle. The exercises I provide have been proven to activate this muscle according to EMG (electromyogram) and ultrasound studies. You will also learn how to continue to progress with the exercises and work with them over time to insure steady gains. Finally, I will outline a simple maintenance program to help you keep fit for years to come.

◉ This book shows you how to treat a possible *cause* of your low-back pain, not merely its symptoms. Since the multifidus contains sensory nerves that report pain, it can surely be a direct source of pain in and of itself. On the other hand, the multifidus also has great potential to indirectly cause back pain when something (perhaps a slipped disc or an unstable vertebra) impairs the multifidus' ability to stabilize the spine properly, which in turn allows other back structures to be abnormally stressed and become painful. Whatever your actual case may be, this we know for certain: *Much solid research has clearly demonstrated a very strong link between abnormal multifidus muscles and low-back pain, and exercising this muscle helps.* Books that teach exercises and techniques that treat symptoms and not causes only show you how to cope with your back problem, and not eliminate it. For instance, massage techniques, using heat, and doing stretching exercises no doubt make many people with back pain feel better temporarily, but really do very little to treat the actual problem and relieve pain over the long run. Be aware, too, that multifidus strengthening exercises not only aim to treat possible direct and indirect causes of your back pain, but also treat its function by improving muscular performance. By learning to restore your spine's function back to normal with the exercises in this book, you will start to shift your focus and energy onto getting better.

It may surprise you, but for just about anything you can name that is thought to be a major source of low-back pain, I can more than likely show you a study that demonstrates it to be present in a person with no back pain at all. A few examples follow.

Most people believe that if a spinal nerve in the low back is being compressed by a disk or bony spur, pain will result. Yet, if this is true, how come a study done once on people with *no back pain* found that a whopping 24 percent of them had spinal nerve compression? Or how about the study that took people with no back pain whatsoever, scanned them with an MRI (magnetic resonance imaging device), and found that a staggering 64 percent of them had abnormal disks? Degenerative disk disease is another finding often blamed for someone's low-back pain, but then again cadaver studies have proven that the disk really begins "degenerating" when we're in our twenties.

I could continue with many more examples, all from well-done clinical studies on people with no low-back pain that have been published in well-respected, peer-reviewed journals over the years, but I think I've made my point. Things such as having one leg longer than another, poor back flexibility, an increased curve in your lower back, or even having the famous "herniated disk" pressing on a nerve in your back are not *necessarily* the cause of your pain. This is simply because researchers can find these things significantly present all too often in people who have absolutely no pain.

It is due to this lack of strong association between these things and back pain that I decided to write a book about the multifidus muscle. Problems with this muscle have been found to exist in many people who carry traditional back pain diagnoses, such as herniated disk, spondylolisthesis, "acute" back pain, "chronic" back pain, and for even individuals who have had low-back surgery. On the other hand, there is no abundance of literature that I know of that shows abnormal problems with the multifidus muscle occurring in people with no back pain. At last the literature is beginning to shed some light on a physical finding (problems with the multifidus) that is present in people with low-back pain but not to any significant degree in a person without pain. The best news of all, however, is that there are also emerging some well-done, randomized, controlled trials that have proven multifidus problems can be treated and corrected with the right kind of exercise.

To say the least, I'm excited and very happy to share this information with you. However, I want to make it perfectly clear from the get-go that doing the multifidus strengthening exercises in this book may not be a cure-all in and of itself for everybody's back pain. Indeed, you may gain varied results. Often times back pain can be a multidimensional problem. And as logic has it, a problem with many dimensions often requires more than one treatment strategy. On the flip side, though, whatever your case may be, I have treated few backs that have failed to gain some benefit from strengthened multifidus muscles. Maybe, then, treating the multifidus will prove to be one important piece of the puzzle.

At the very minimum, you will become a better-informed consumer by reading this book. As I discuss the research and literature related to the multifidus, I will also be showing you how to tell effective back-pain treatments from less effective ones before you invest the time, money, and energy in them. Also included is a question-and-answer section, as well as a list of other treatments for low-back pain that have been proven effective in randomized controlled trials—yet other options for your consideration that you might not have known about, all completely backed by good clinical trials.

There truly is something for every back-pain sufferer to gain from this book, whether it's pain relief through the exercises or education about your back pain and its treatment. I've intentionally kept this book short so you can get the information you need quickly and can begin the exercises as soon as possible. Please remember, though, that knowledge is power, so make sure that you read the entire book as each chapter will contribute to your education about your back problem and make you an overall better-informed consumer.

Before I close, I'd like to congratulate you on the giant step you've just taken. By seeking answers through reading this book, you're taking an active approach in your health care and getting even closer to solving your back pain troubles. For that, you have my respect.

—Jim Johnson, P.T.

No problem can withstand the assault of sustained thinking.
—Voltaire

1

What's a Multifidus?

It is not the answer that enlightens, but the question.

—Eugene Ionesco

"A multi-whatafus?" said a patient one time during an office visit.

"Multifidus," I replied. "It's a group of muscles in your low back. They're doing a lot of research on it now and finding out that people with back pain often have problems with this muscle."

The patient then looked at me a little less confused and said, "Oh."

This is the normal response I get when I start talking about the multifidus (pronounced "mull-TIFF-i-dus"). If you've never heard of it, don't feel alone. Most medical professionals, including many doctors I have treated, also look perplexed when I mention the multifidus. To be completely honest, the multifidus wasn't significant to me either until after I had graduated from physical therapy school and started specializing in low-back problems. Since the multifidus is probably a mystery muscle to most people,

I think it's best to start out by briefly reviewing what it is, where it is, how to find it, and what exactly it does.

A Note on Terminology

While the multifidus is really a group of muscles, it's referred to in the back literature in the singular. So, before we start, you should know that I'll be calling it "the multifidus" unless I'm talking about its anatomy.

The Multifidus

The multifidus is one of your many back muscles. The name comes from the Latin words *multus*, meaning many, and *findo*, to cleave. You can see from the picture of the multifidus muscles (Figure 1) how early anatomists might come up with that name for this muscle.

Back muscles are arranged on the spine in several layers, with the multifidus being one of the more deeply situated ones. The multifidus muscle group starts out in the lower back and runs the entire length of the spine, all the way up to the neck. However, it is not just one big muscle that runs all the way from the top to the bottom. Instead, it takes many individual multifidus muscles combined, each crossing two to five levels of vertebrae, to cover the entire spinal column. In this way, the multifidus is capable of gaining fine control over just a single segment of the spine. This anatomic detail is important to remember when we discuss back problems later in the book. Researchers are now finding out that in some people with low-back pain, it's not always the whole multifidus muscle group that is the problem. In many cases, it's just a *single* multifidus muscle at only one level of the spine that's not working properly.

All muscles need nerves to carry a signal to them, making them contract and relax. Think of a nerve as like an electrical cord that carries power to a lamp to make it light up. The multifidus is no different in that it also needs nerves to function. What does make it different from all the other back muscles is that each multifidus muscle gets its nerve messages from only *one* level of the spinal cord. Anatomists call this being *segmentally innervated*. What this means to the multifidus muscle is that it can be more prone to having problems. Other back muscles have their nerves or "electrical cords" coming from several different levels of the spine to power them, so that if one nerve doesn't work well, it still has the others to help it out. The multifidus doesn't have it so easy, however, as its nerve supply comes from just a single level of the spine. If something goes wrong at a certain level in the spine, such as a slipped disk pressing on a nerve, a single multifidus muscle could be in trouble without a backup.

Another interesting anatomic fact about the multifidus is that it's connected to each of the small joints in your spine, also known as the *facet joints* (see Figure 1). It does this by way of its attachment directly to the joint capsule (the tissue that surrounds each of the facet joints). This is significant for the spine's function, as the multifidus can exert a pull on this capsule and prevent it from becoming caught inside the joint as you move your back throughout the day. One can already begin to see, just by this short discussion of anatomy alone, how a multifidus not doing its job properly has great potential to create a low-back problem.

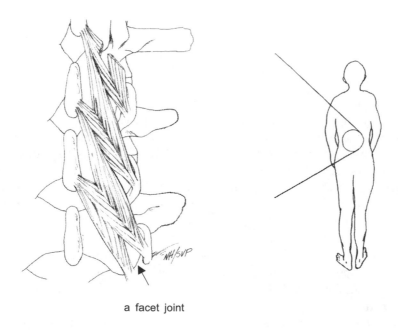

a facet joint

Figure 1. Drawing of multifidus muscle courtesy of Stanley Paris, Ph.D., P.T.

Finding the Multifidus Muscle on Yourself

The multifidus muscle extends along the entire length of the spine, but is much thicker in the low-back region at your waist level. It is here where you will be able to palpate (feel) it directly through the overlying skin the best. To do this, you must first locate the bones that stick up in the center of your back. These are called the *spinous processes* and are easily felt, as they are the only ones that stick out in the middle and run up your whole back. Once you have felt these bones, feel directly off to the side of one of them in your low back (either side will do), and you should feel a soft mass of tissue. These are some of your lower-back multifidus muscles. They sit nicely in a groove on each side of the spinous process bones that stick up. As you move farther up the spine, it becomes harder to feel just the multifidus muscle alone. This is because the muscles of the back are arranged in layers. As you feel your way up toward the head from waist level, the other back muscles will soon begin to overlap and cover up the multifidus. This in effect buries the multifidus at higher levels of the back, making it less accessible and impossible to feel in isolation. You can be confident, however, that you are feeling *just* the multifidus muscle under the skin at the beltline level in your lower-back area.

You now know more about finding the multifidus muscle than many medical professionals and most physical-therapy students. Take a moment now to feel the multifidus muscles in your own low back. Normal muscles usually feel soft, almost spongy. Your fingers should be able to go quite easily through the overlying skin and superficial fat, sinking down into the muscle tissue without the sensation of hard resistance. Additionally, normal muscles need a certain amount of side-to-side play (or *excursion*). This is because as your muscles contract, they naturally shorten and widen a bit making this side-to-side motion something necessary for proper functioning. You can check this out by pushing the multifidus sideways (horizontally) and feeling for its willingness to move and give.

Muscles that are overworked or irritated for one reason or another can sometimes go into spasm, feeling firm or even very hard. When patients come to see me, they will often times describe their back muscles by saying that they feel "knots" in their back. These kinds of things will limit the overall function of a muscle, making its job harder or even impossible to do. Remember that a little tenderness here and there is okay, depending on how hard you're pressing, but no muscle should really be that painful in its normal state. If you do feel a lot of tenderness or perhaps some pain, this could possibly signal that there is a problem with your multifidus muscle.

What a Multifidus Muscle Does

So what exactly does a funny looking muscle like the multifidus do anyway? To answer this question, I found that I had to look at two rather specific areas in order to get a whole and complete picture of its job in the back. The first is the study of kinesiology, where one looks at things such as the angle that a muscle can pull on a bone. The other area deals with what is known as electromyography or in medical parlance, EMG. EMG's look at how active the muscle is during certain movements of the spine. Let's take a brief look at each without getting too bogged down in scientific details.

The Kinesiology of the Multifidus

Don't be alarmed by the word "kinesiology." It's just a big word somebody made up a long time ago that means the study of how things move. Now that wasn't as bad as it sounded, was it? You can see from this definition that we do need to know a little about kinesiology in order to fully appreciate what this interesting muscle really does.

Think of muscles like rubber bands that are stretched from one bone to another in your body. When muscles receive a signal by the nerves to contract, they then pull on the bones they're attached to, and like a stretched rubber band, they become shorter in length. This then causes the bone that the muscle is pulling on to move. It's in this manner that we are able to move our bones, and in turn, our arms and legs. Now that we have this knowledge, we can use it to figure out what the job of the multifidus is in the back.

You can see from the picture of the multifidus (Figure 1) that it attaches on the backside of the vertebrae in your spine. This clue tells us that the muscle pulls the vertebrae or spine backwards, since a rubber band stretched this way over the back of two bones could only pull them in this direction. Therefore, just by looking at where the muscle is placed in the back and the direction that it pulls, one can see that *the multifidus is responsible for a backward tilting effect on each of the individual vertebrae that make up the spine.*

Electromyography and the Multifidus

We now know what the multifidus can do as it pulls on two vertebrae bones in your back. However, this does not really tell the whole story of what its job is. Sure, we know that it pulls the vertebrae backwards, but when does it do this and with what motions? This is where the study of electromyography or EMG comes in quite handy.

An EMG study starts when a muscle is hooked up to a machine that can tell us when the muscle is active and working. The machine can do this by recording the electrical activity of the muscles as one uses them. When I first started studying the multifidus, I went straight to the medical library to find all the research articles I could get my hands on that studied the multifidus muscle with EMG machine. I was glad to find that there was indeed much literature published in medical journals through the years that had studied the back muscles with an EMG machine as people performed certain movements or exercises. I found the following to be true from a compilation of all the available studies. Your multifidus *is* active and working when you are:

- ◉ standing still
- ◉ bending forward
- ◉ twisting to either side
- ◉ picking or lifting things up
- ◉ walking

Your multifidus is *not* active or working when you are:

- ◉ sidebending the back directly to the left or right
- ◉ bending backwards when there is no resistance
- ◉ laying down

Keep in mind that this information comes from studies that were done in persons *without* back pain. This is to say that the above is what occurs normally. Some back conditions may cause the multifidus to contract poorly, continuously, or with activities and motions it isn't normally active in.

You can see from the above list that the multifidus is a very busy muscle in the back. The available research indicates that this muscle is involved in the vast majority of movements and activities that we do with our spines every day. But hold on a minute—didn't we just look at the kinesiology of the multifidus and find that all it does is pull the vertebrae backwards in a rocking type motion? Indeed it does, but obviously this motion is very important while the spine is moving in various ways. Otherwise, it would not be as highly active as it is with so many back motions.

Summary

After reading this chapter, you can begin to gain a little appreciation for this little-known muscle and also begin to see its importance in the overall functioning of the back. The next chapter will show you exactly what sets the multifidus apart from the other back muscles and why it is so special. I will also cover problems that back researchers are only now beginning to find with this muscle in people who suffer with low-back pain. But before we proceed, I've provided a short list of the most important information from this chapter to use as a handy reference. Please take a moment and briefly review it, as we will also be using this knowledge as we move through each section of the book.

Key Points

- The multifidus is a deep back muscle.

- Your back has many individual multifidus muscles that, when combined, run the entire length of your spine.

- The multifidus muscle is capable of controlling the motions of individual vertebrae in your spine.

- Nerves that make the multifidus work come from just one segment of the spine, unlike other back muscles which get their nerves from several different segments, helping to protect their function.

- The multifidus muscle attaches directly to the joints in your spine.

- The multifidus can be easily felt in isolation in the *lower* back region.

- A normal muscle is not painful to the touch—your multifidus shouldn't be either.

- The multifidus is a highly active muscle in the back that is involved in many everyday motions and activities.

2

What Makes the Multifidus So Special?

My patient, Ruby, leaned slightly forward in her chair, becoming more curious by the minute. She had been suffering from back pain for many years, had seen countless professionals, and had yet to hear about this multifidus muscle. "This isn't the only muscle in my back, right?" she said.

"Oh no," I replied. "There are many others, and they have funny names too."

"Then what makes this muscle so special?" Ruby asked.

"That's a very good question," I said. "There are some very big differences that back researchers have found that make this muscle the most important one in your back."

I then pointed to a skeleton of the spine and said, "Let me explain."

I always admire the skeptical patient and wish there were more of them. Patients should never just accept whatever they are told if a treatment or diagnosis isn't really clear to them just because a medical professional told them it was so. Ruby asked a very good question, "What makes the multifidus so special?" It can be frightening to be a consumer going through the health-care system with back pain. As if it isn't already enough that patients have to deal with things such as unintelligible medical terms and insurance hassles, it seems like everybody has a different explanation of why your back hurts and has a different treatment to offer. So what's a patient to do?

Ten years ago, when I first started out treating back pain, I encountered similar problems. If you think that it's confusing for a patient, I can tell you that it can be equally challenging for the medical professional. For instance, ask two therapists how long they have their patients hold a stretch to lengthen a muscle and you'll likely get two completely different answers. And that's just something as simple as stretching, let alone getting an agreement on something more complex such as what's causing a patient's back pain.

As a physical therapist, it was these constant inconsistencies between medical professionals that frustrated me no end—how long to hold a stretch, the number of sets of an exercise to strengthen a muscle, or coming up with same patient diagnosis. As my aggravation grew, I began thinking that since medicine had been studying back pain for decades, we surely must have *some* definitive answers by now. Maybe by falling back on the scientific literature and getting "just the facts" we could all be on the same page when dealing with this complex problem of back pain. This is exactly what the intention of this next section is—to present only facts from the scientific literature that will show you exactly why I have chosen to tell you about the multifidus and not some other back muscle.

Anatomical Differences

The branch of science called *anatomy* is simply the study of the structure of things or how they are arranged in the body. For instance, the fact that you have five fingers or that the heart is on the left side of your body is due to your anatomy. Yes, researchers do find subtle variations sometimes from person to person, but for the most part, we're really all quite similar.

I have already discussed the basic anatomy of the multifidus in the first chapter (didn't know you had been studying anatomy, did you?). However, since there are extremely important distinctions that set the multifidus apart from other back muscles, I'll go over them in a little bit more detail here.

Segmentally Innervated

The multifidus, like all muscles, needs a nerve (remember, like an electrical cord) to carry a signal to it. It's this signal that makes the muscle contract and work. The nerves that go to the back muscles all branch off from a cluster of important nerves (the spinal cord) that are housed inside the vertebrae. The vertebrae, or your "back bones" as most know them, are stacked like blocks, one upon another to make up your spine. This stacking, in effect, creates different "levels" in the back.

In order to make talking about the back and its structures easier, anatomists gave the different bones and levels names. For instance, did you know that your low back (or in medical terms, *lumbar spine*) was made up of only five vertebrae? It follows then that the first *lumbar* (low back) vertebra is called "L-1," the second lumbar vertebra "L-2," and so on. Pretty easy, huh?

Now to get to the point of all this: Anatomists named the spinal nerves of the back after the level at which they come off the spinal cord. So, the spinal nerve that comes out between the L-2 and L-3 vertebrae, for instance, is known as the L-2 nerve. The nerve that comes out from between the L-3 and L-4 vertebrae is called the L-3 nerve. Now you can see what I mean about the nerves coming from different levels of the spine. Just keep thinking of the back as a bunch of stacked blocks (the vertebrae) creating different levels. In between these blocks emerge the spinal nerves that have come straight from the spinal cord.

Unfortunately for the multifidus, it does not have nerves from different levels of the spine to make it contract and work. Each multifidus has nerve supply from just a single level of the spine that it depends on. This is what we referred to earlier as *segmental innervation*. As an example, a multifidus at the L-4 and L-5 vertebra level gets its supply from just the L-4 nerve only. Other back muscles at that same area might get their supply from the L-4 as well as the L-5 nerve.

So what does this mean to our favorite back muscle? It means simply that it has no backup nerves like the other back muscles do. Each multifidus depends on its single spinal nerve supply to make it contract. If something presses on its only spinal nerve, it's in trouble, unlike other back muscles that have several spinal nerves supplying it. This anatomical fact perfectly explains why researchers are in many cases finding problems with just one multifidus muscle at a single level of the spine in back pain patients. The multifidus is indeed more prone to having problems due to its segmental innervation. This is one anatomical reason that makes the multifidus so unique.

Attachment to the Joints

The multifidus muscle has several attachments to the vertebrae, one being to the little joints in the spine. Remember that the vertebrae are like blocks stacked on one another. As the top half of one vertebrae comes together with the bottom half of another one, they create a little joint, one on each side, that we call *the facet joint* (I have no idea where they get these names from). It's pronounced "FAH-set," in case you're wondering.

Around this facet joint (like every other joint in the body) is tissue called the joint capsule. It is on to this capsule that part of the multifidus muscle attaches itself. This would not be such a big deal in and of itself except that parts of the capsule continue into the edges around the facet joints. It's part of the job of the multifidus to contract with certain back movements and help pull the capsule away from the joint so it won't be nipped. A multifidus that isn't working properly has the potential to allow this capsule to be pinched by the joint. Since it's an anatomical fact that the capsule has nerve endings, any pinching of it can result in an attack of back pain. This might help explain some of the strange cases of acute back-pain attacks people complain of after doing seemingly simple motions that they do every day, such as sweeping a floor. If the joint is caught off guard and the multifidus muscle is unable to control things—ouch!

A Proven Stabilizer of the Back

Having good stability in your back means that the back is able to keep itself in positions that are safe. When the back loses this control, even momentarily, motion can take place in positions that may potentially cause damage to its structures. For example, say you're putting a dish away on a high shelf, a little to the right side, which causes you to stretch and slightly twist the low back. The back that has good stability will be able to keep its vertebrae, joints, and disks within a safe zone and be able to control its motion well. Additionally, it has the ability to hold odd positions better for a longer period of time. On the other hand, a back that has poor stability is unable to control motion well and could let the spine exceed its zone of safety—thereby risking injury.

The spine has several ways to keep itself stable:

◉ With "passive" structures such as the ligaments, joints, bones, etc.

◉ With the muscles that actively contract

While these elements do contribute to the stability of the back, some things have been shown to provide more support than others. Research on back stabilization has demonstrated that the human spinal column without muscles is unable to support the normal loads that are placed on it during everyday activities. This tells us that just the passive structures like ligaments, bones, and disks are in and of themselves quite incapable of supporting the spine. The muscles stand out as a major source of stability for our backs.

So now that we know that the muscles play a crucial role in back stability, we need to know which ones are the most important so that we can specifically train and strengthen them. While all the muscles in the low back have the ability to support and stabilize the spine to some degree, guess which one has emerged from the research as being able to contribute more to the stability of the spine than the other back muscles? You guessed it—the multifidus! Here are several facts that the current research has uncovered about the multifidus that pinpoints it as being a key stabilizer of the spine:

◉ The multifidus muscle is capable of providing control over individual segments of the spine.

◉ When it contracts, the multifidus can stiffen the vertebrae and, in turn, the individual levels of the spine, thereby providing support and stability.

◉ About two-thirds of the total stiffness that all the back muscles can provide for support through muscle contraction comes from the multifidus muscle.

A healthy back is one that has good support and can keep itself from being injured. As you can see, the spine relies quite heavily on its muscles for this job. Of all the muscles in the back, the research identifies the multifidus muscle as having the biggest role of all in providing this necessary stability and control.

Identifying the Problem

When back researchers study the spine in hopes of identifying a source of back pain, one thing they do is look for differences between those people who have back pain and those who are pain-free. By looking for such differences between a healthy back and a painful one, researchers are hoping that an association can be made and a cause found. For example, let's say a researcher studies ten people with back pain and ten people without back pain. He then takes an X ray of all twenty people's spines and looks for any differences between the healthy backs and the painful ones. If the ten people with back pain all have slipped disks, for example, and none of the pain-free backs do, it might be assumed then that the slipped disks are the source of the back pain.

If only it were always this simple. Take depression for example. Many studies have identified depression in people who suffer from chronic low-back pain. The problem with these studies is that we don't know which came first, the back pain or the depression. Maybe initial depression caused the back pain, or maybe the people became depressed because they already had back pain. It's the old chicken-and-egg thing.

While such problems continue to cause gray areas in back-pain research, there are epidemiological studies that have looked at associations between certain factors and back pain. Here are a few that have been shown *not* to be associated with back pain. The list may surprise you.

- ◉ How much you weigh
- ◉ How tall you are
- ◉ Having one leg longer than the other
- ◉ Having scoliosis (except in back curves of 80 degrees or more)
- ◉ The curve of your low back (doesn't matter if it's flat or you have an increased curve)

⊙ The flexibility of your low back

⊙ Having one hip higher than the other

Interesting, huh? For further, detailed reading, check out the reference section in the back of the book. Now let's look at a list of how common some of these so-called "abnormalities" in your low back are, as well as some X ray findings and their association with pain.

Here are some X ray findings that have *no association* with nonspecific low-back pain:

⊙ Spondylolisthesis

⊙ Spondylolysis

⊙ Spina bifida

⊙ Transitional vertebrae

⊙ Spondylosis

⊙ Schuermann's disease

And now consider these percentages of structural "abnormalities" that have been found in studies on people with *pain-free* backs:

⊙ The percentage of people who have compressed nerves and no back pain is 24 percent with a myelogram test.

⊙ Sixty-four percent of people who report no back pain show abnormal disks with an MRI exam.

⊙ A CAT scan will show spinal stenosis (narrowing of the holes where nerves pass through) in 3 percent of persons without back pain.

⊙ Degeneration of the facet joints can be found on MRI exams in 8 percent of asymptomatic spines.

Remember that the above shows the percentage of these abnormalities that are present in persons with *no* low-back pain! As an example from the above, if you took a hundred people with no back pain, approximately sixty-four of them are walking around with disk abnormalities (such as herniated or "slipped disks"), eight of them show degeneration of the joints in the spine, and so on. Taking the above information as a whole, it would appear that many structural abnormalities can have very little to do with a person's low-back pain. Furthermore, there are many people that have such "abnormalities" and live every day without pain.

The main point of all this is to show you that just because something abnormal is found on an X ray or appears asymmetrical on a physical examination, this does not automatically make it the cause of the back pain. After reading much clinical literature on backs, it became apparent to me that just about any abnormal physical finding I could name that I thought was responsible for a patient's low-back pain could also be found in individuals with no pain at all. Now don't get me wrong—this does not mean that a structural abnormality can *never* be a cause of a person's back pain. There are instances where it's obviously a clear-cut source of pain. Take a "slipped disk" for example. Of course a disk can bulge and press on a nerve and produce back and leg pain. And if this is truly what's going on, it should not only be apparent on a radiographic test such as an MRI, but the patient should also show neurological signs (such as a decrease in reflexes, strength, or sensation) that correspond exactly to the nerve that is being pressed on by the disk. In reality, this perfect picture is seen in only a minority of cases. Such strong correlations between physical exams and patient's symptoms are few and far between in clinical practice. Any medical professional who has treated back pain would probably tend to agree.

This puzzle brings us back to the subject of this book, the multifidus. As I said earlier, just about any abnormal structural finding that is cited as a cause of low-back pain can be shown to be present in significant percentages of people without low-back pain. This discrepancy is what caught my attention the most when I started reading the research about the multifidus muscle. My first reaction was, "Oh boy, so here's another so-called abnormality that we will probably later find out is present in many asymptomatic people." To date, though, this has not been the case. Abnormalities of the multifidus have been hard to find in pain-free individuals to any large degree. Here's a case in point. A study came out in *Spine* in 1995 where a researcher named Haig and coworkers looked specifically for any abnormalities of the low-back muscles in persons free of low-back pain. Using quantified needle electromyography (a type of EMG test that uses needles), they examined thirty-five individuals. Their conclusion? Normal people have few, if any electromyographic abnormalities in their low-back muscles. Stein (1993) also found the same to be true in his subjects without back pain. And that's just looking at the multifidus people with no back pain using one diagnostic device. When researchers take tissue samples from people with no back pain and examine them under a microscope, only around 1 to 5 percent at most have ever been found to be abnormal. Yes, this does show us that there are a few individuals walking around with no back pain and a multifidus abnormality. This we need to be keenly aware of. However, when one compares something like multifidus structural abnormalities (1 to 5 percent) to the prevalence of other commonly cited causes of back pain such as the disk (64 percent of people with no back pain having abnormal disks on MRI) or compressed nerves (24 percent free of pain showing nerve compression on CT myelograms), it does tend to put things in perspective. As with my physical-therapy students that I teach, I highly encourage you to draw your own conclusions from the available data. However, it seems reasonable to assume at this time that there are actually very few people indeed who have no back pain and an abnormal multifidus muscle.

Over time, more studies will accumulate and begin to shed even more light on the very distinct differences that exist between the multifidus muscles in healthy backs versus painful ones. Let's have a brief look now at what the latest studies reveal about the abnormalities researchers have pinpointed with the multifidus muscle in patients with many different types of low- back problems.

The Multifidus Muscle and Specific Structural Problems

Herniated Disks

The disk is a structure that sits between the stacked vertebrae that make up your spine. It has several functions, an important one being to act as a shock absorber. Think of the disks like little jelly doughnuts. Inside the disk is a jelly-like substance that can attract water, thus giving it a better ability to absorb forces. Interestingly, studies show that we are actually taller in the morning than we are at night. This is due to the disk being able to increase its size at night by pulling in water more effectively as we take the pressure off our backs. Then when we get out of bed in the morning and begin to vertically load our spines (standing and sitting upright), fluid is forced from the disks throughout the day, and we become a bit shorter by nighttime.

Many people have heard of a "slipped disk." This term, however, does not accurately describe the problem that really occurs with the disk. In reality, the disk is anchored firmly between two vertebrae and cannot "slip" out. What usually happens, however, is the jelly-like center of the disk (called the *nucleus pulposus*) can be forced out of its place and usually begins to work its way out the back of the disk. Medically, this is called a *disk herniation*, due to the jelly substance herniating out of the center and toward the back of the disk. This would not be a big deal, except that we have spinal nerves passing right next to the disks. A disk herniation then becomes a problem when the jelly-like substance presses directly against one of these irritated spinal nerves. Most people know this problem as a "pinched nerve."

While medicine has known for years that a disk pressing on an irritated spinal nerve is capable of causing back and leg pain, it hasn't been until recently that its effect on the back muscles has been studied. The following is a summary of the changes that have been found to take place in the multifidus muscle in patients with a confirmed herniated disk.

- ◉ A herniated disk causes the multifidus to be overactive and contract more often than it should.

- ◉ Biopsies taken during surgery for disk herniations have shown that the multifidus has much smaller muscle fibers than normal (mainly the fast twitch kind—those muscle fibers that contract the quickest).

Apparently, disk herniations take their toll on structures other than just the classic "pinched nerve" as had been previously thought. The research has yet to tell us why the above changes can occur with a herniated disk, nor is it able to pinpoint exact causes. However, it is interesting to note that studies including back muscle exercises to treat patients with herniated disks have shown high success rates. More on that later.

Pregnancy

Low-back pain is an extremely common complaint during pregnancy. It's natural then that researchers would sooner or later get around to studying the multifidus muscle during pregnancy (unfortunately, the majority of back researchers are men, or it probably would have been sooner).

To conduct these studies, researchers have used the EMG (electromyography—a test that looks at how active the muscle is by measuring its electrical activity). In a 1998 study in the journal *Archives of Physical Medicine and Rehabilitation,* Sihvonen and coworkers hooked pregnant participants to an EMG machine and examined the response of the multifidus muscle as the women bent forward and returned upright.

The normal response of your multifidus muscle to such a task is for it to contract as you lower your trunk down and bend over. Then, at around 40 to 70 degrees of bending forward, the back muscles normally relax. The exact reason for this is not known, but one theory is that the ligaments take over at some point and since the muscles are no longer needed, they relax. An example of this motion would be when you are bending down to pick something up off the floor. The multifidus works to lower you down until about 40 to 70 degrees and then suddenly relaxes. The following is what the study on pregnant women found when they were asked to bend forward with EMG monitoring and rate their pain intensity at various weeks into pregnancy:

◉ Increased multifidus muscle activity correlated with the intensity of the back pain that was felt during pregnancy.

◉ Increased multifidus muscle activity predicted which females, initially free of pain at the beginning of the study, would eventually get low-back pain during their pregnancy.

So it seems that the multifidus muscle can be affected during pregnancy as well. Apparently, in some cases the multifidus keeps continuously contracting during certain motions (like bending and picking things up) when it should be relaxing. Why this occurs is not known; however, this abnormal pattern does match the intensity of pain one will have during pregnancy as well as having the ability to predict who will have low-back pain.

The Multifidus after Back Surgery

Many studies have looked at the state of the multifidus muscle in patients who have undergone various back procedures. Upon reviewing these studies, I have found that they can be divided into two categories. There are those studies that look with EMGs at the function of the multifidus, and others that look at the actual structure of the muscle under a microscope. Let's take a brief look at the findings of both. Some common structural and EMG changes found in the multifidus muscle of patients after back surgery include:

- The muscle fibers are smaller than normal, specifically the "fast-twitch" fibers.

- Changes are present in the inner structure of the muscle fibers.

- Long-lasting denervation (loss of nerve supply) of the multifidus is frequently seen.

Surgery is certainly effective at removing the disk material that is pressing on the nerve. However, in order to get to the nerve and disk, the back muscles must be pulled or *retracted* off to the sides while another surgeon removes the disk. Generally speaking, the longer the surgery takes, the longer the retraction time, meaning more trauma to the tissues. Studies that have examined the back muscles after surgery suggest several reasons why these changes above occur. One is simply the pressure exerted by the retraction tool itself that can cause direct injury to the muscle fibers, damage that's compounded the longer the tool is in place. Another reason is the fact that while muscle is retracted, blood flow is necessarily slowed to that muscle, resulting in more damage.

Now that you know that these changes more than likely take place with most back surgeries, you may wonder how this affects the outcome of those surgeries. Can the muscle recover over time? Several studies have examined the relationship between the outcome of the surgery and the functioning of the multifidus muscle. Interestingly enough, when patients are placed in either a positive or negative outcome group, those who have done poorly have more muscle wasting and pathologic changes in their multifidus muscles than the positive-outcome group.

Spondylolisthesis and Instability

If you thought the word multifidus was hard to pronounce, try this next one. *Spondylolisthesis* (pronounced "SPON-duh-low-lis-THEE-sis") is a condition where one vertebra has slipped in relation to another. The classic example is a vertebra slipping in a forward direction (like toward your belly button) on the one below it. There are several reasons why this can occur. The most common one is a crack in the bone between the two joints that connect the vertebra. When this happens, the vertebra has less support holding it in place and therefore more of a tendency to slip. A spondylolisthesis is usually graded on a scale of I through IV, with a grade I meaning that the vertebra has slipped 25 percent on the vertebra below, grade II a 50 percent slip, and so on.

Spine surgeons look for a spondylolisthesis in particular as a potential source of back pain. It is thought that when a vertebra has slipped forward, it could be unstable and thus cause pain due to the excessive motion that puts increased tension on the tissues. The treatment in such a case is to fuse the two vertebrae together, usually with bone taken from the hip, to stabilize the segment. Hopefully, painful symptoms are then alleviated as the vertebra is stabilized and cannot cause further problems.

There are, of course, many reasons for a vertebra to become unstable. Degenerative changes that happen due to injury or old age are often blamed. Joints and ligaments can become slack, causing increased motion in the vertebra. But whatever the cause, increased motion can be measured radiographically (with an X-ray), and a diagnosis of *instability* is usually given if the medical professional feels that the vertebra has more motion than it should.

With spondylolisthesis and instability having gained much attention as potential sources of back pain, it's no wonder that researchers wanted to study the multifidus in patients with such conditions. When I searched the literature to write this section, I was unable to locate any studies thus far that examined the multifidus specifically in spondylolisthesis patients. However, I was able to find good research that studied patients with *hypermobile* vertebrae in their backs (vertebrae that have more motion than normal), as determined with X rays. These patients were then further examined with EMG studies. The following are some of the major findings from the literature. Some changes in the multifidus muscle found in patients with hypermobile vertebrae included:

☉ Abnormal EMGs of the multifidus muscle correlate well with vertebrae that have excessive motion. In other words, abnormality in the multifidus can be an indication that there is too much motion in the vertebrae. In many patients, it is only the multifidus muscle just at the level of the hypermobile vertebrae that is abnormal.

☉ Decreased EMG activity is found in the multifidus muscle when patients were asked to perform activities that make it contract.

◉ Research has shown that abnormal EMG signals can improve in patients with hypermobile vertebrae after having them complete exercise programs that include strengthening the multifidus muscle.

◉ Significantly reduced pain and disability have been documented in patients with confirmed spondylolisthesis (slipped vertebrae) after completing an exercise program that specifically strengthens the multifidus muscle.

Earlier in this chapter, we discussed that the spine relies quite heavily on the back muscles for its support. Of these muscles, the research has pinpointed the multifidus as playing a key role. It comes as no surprise then that when the back is having difficulty with stability, as with the case of a hypermobile vertebra, we can demonstrate problems with the multifidus as well.

Changes in the Multifidus in Patients with Back Pain

Classifying the Patients

One commonly used way of classifying back pain is by the length of time it has been present. The following is a frequently seen system used in the scientific back research, and many patients referred to me for physical therapy have been diagnosed with one of these as well. See which category you might fit into.

◉ *Acute back pain.* Start of back pain up to six weeks

◉ *Subacute back pain.* Back pain from six weeks up to three months

◉ *Chronic back pain.* Having back pain at least three months

As an example of using the above classification system, say you just hurt your back lifting a heavy box this morning. That would be called *acute* back pain. If the pain continued for two months, it would be *subacute* back pain. If you were unfortunate and continued to have pain for longer than three months duration, you would be suffering with *chronic* back pain.

It's very important to know where you fall on this timeline scheme of low-back pain. Most studies that test the effectiveness of a certain treatment for low-back pain classify patients in the study using these guidelines. By knowing what kind of low-back pain the treatment is effective for, you can determine which ones will work best for you. For example, if you hear about magnets helping relieve low-back pain, you will certainly want to find out if they tested the treatment on acute or chronic back-pain patients. Believe me, it makes a big difference. Some treatments for back pain have been shown to work better on chronic back pain than acute, or vice versa. Manipulation (or the skilled, passive movement of a joint, like when a chiropractor cracks your back) is one such example. Strong evidence exists for the effectiveness of manipulation for chronic low-back pain, but not as much for acute. So, the next time someone tells you that they know of a treatment that is effective for low-back pain, ask them what type.

Now that you know the difference between acute, subacute, and chronic low-back pain, we will talk about what the research on the multifidus has found using these categories. I will discuss acute and subacute back pain together, as this is how it's presented in the research. Here are the pertinent facts on each from the back research for acute and subacute back-pain patients.

- Using ultrasound techniques, the multifidus muscle has been shown to be smaller on just *one side* of the back in patients with acute and subacute low-back pain.

- The side of the back with the smaller multifidus muscle matches the exact same side as the patient's pain.

- Muscle wasting occurs at just a *single* vertebral level in the majority of patients with acute and subacute back pain.

- This muscle wasting, as seen on ultrasound, does *not* automatically recover over time, even as symptoms resolve.

- Strengthening exercises cause the multifidus muscle to recover more quickly and more completely after back pain than it normally would.

The changes documented in the multifidus muscle above come from studies where most patients had no specific diagnosis. This means that no obvious source of pain could be identified, yet the researchers who were looking specifically for problems with the multifidus found some very interesting results. What's equally notable is that the researchers didn't find just some general changes in the back muscles, they found specific muscle wasting of the multifidus muscle on just *one side* of the back that perfectly matched the painful side. Also note that even though a person's back pain improves, this does not necessarily mean that the multifidus is back to normal. Researchers who follow patients over a period of time have noted that the decreased size of the multifidus does not go back to normal automatically just because the back pain was resolved. Finally, it's encouraging that doing strengthening exercises can help the multifidus return to its normal state.

That's about it for acute and subacute back pain, so we'll move on now to the information researchers have found in patients suffering from chronic low-back pain.

- There is a significant correlation between multifidus muscle wasting and the complaints of leg pain.

- MRI tests reveal that chronic low-back pain patients have smaller multifidus muscles than healthy control subjects.

- Exercise has been documented to increase both the size and the strength of the multifidus muscle in patients with chronic back pain.

- Abnormal EMGs have been consistently observed in the multifidus muscles of chronic back-pain patients, usually at just *one level* of the spine.

- Abnormal EMGs can also return to normal after exercise therapy.

Sound like a broken record? It should. And what's really interesting is that the above information comes from not only many different studies, but from many different researchers as well. These are not merely the findings of one or two researchers who keep drawing the same conclusions over and over no matter what patient population they look at. Certainly it's very noteworthy that no matter who looks at the multifidus muscle and studies it, the same findings keep cropping up.

You will also note that researchers have used many different kinds of tools to try and evaluate the function of the multifidus. MRIs, which use a magnetic field to create detailed pictures of the spine, have sufficient ability to assess for size differences in the muscles. EMGs look at the electrical activity of muscles as the back goes through certain movements. Strength, assessed in various ways, can also be quantified and compared to known nor-mal values of back-muscle strength. And then there's the biopsy, where a tiny incision is made and a piece of back muscle is taken out. Later, this piece of muscle is looked at under a microscope and analyzed for structural changes compared to normal tissues. Indeed, it seems that regardless of what tools researchers have chosen to analyze the multifidus muscle with, the conclusions are all similar.

Summary

After reading this chapter, you should have a good idea as to what makes the multifidus so special. Like the patient in the beginning of this chapter, you need to be aware of the possible role that the multifidus might be playing in your back pain, as well as the rationale behind targeting this particular muscle with exercise therapy. But while I have made a pretty sound argument demonstrating that a majority of low-back pain sufferers with a variety of conditions can have a problem with the multifidus, this does not in and of itself prove that an exercise to strengthen it will cure back pain. The only way to really demonstrate that exer-cising your multifidus helps low-back pain is through carefully controlled clinical trials. And that is what the next chapter is all about.

Key Points

- A back that has good stability can keep itself in safe positions and thereby avoid injury.

- The muscles are a major source of stability for the spine—a human spine without muscles is unable to support normal loads.

- The multifidus can control the individual segments (vertebrae) of your back.

- When back muscles contract, they "stiffen" the spine, thereby stabilizing and protecting it.

- About two-thirds of the total stiffness that the back muscles can produce for support through muscle contraction comes from the multifidus muscle.

- Most structural abnormalities (weight, one leg longer than the other, etc.) actually have very little to do with back pain according to much epidemiological research.

- A high percentage of people *free of back pain* can show a variety of structural abnormalities in the spine on imaging tests like MRIs, X rays, etc.

- In contrast, people free of back pain have few, if any, EMG or structural abnormalities in their multifidus muscles.

- Abnormalities of the multifidus muscle have been found in patients with many different types of low-back problems.

3

The Multifidus and Back Pain: What the Scientific Studies Have to Say

There's a mighty big difference between good, sound reasons and reasons that sound good.

—Hillis

Up to this point, we have covered a lot of information about the multifidus muscle. We have discussed:

- What the multifidus is, where it is, and how you can find it

- What the multifidus muscle does, as well as its critical importance to the spine

- Documented changes in the multifidus muscle found in people with various back conditions and diagnoses

At a glance, all the above seems proof enough to move on to an exercise chapter and begin to exercise. So what's up with this chapter?

Well, great therapies for body aches and pains all start out with information like the kind we've discussed. However, all the facts so far only make a case for exercising the multifidus, providing a heckuva rationale. Unfortunately, all this information doesn't necessarily mean that exercising the multifidus will solve a back problem. To prove this, the scientific community has come up with a tool to provide the highest level of proof that a treatment is truly effective. This is known as the *randomized, controlled trial*.

All right, don't start turning pages now and skipping to the exercise chapter just yet. Action is just around the corner, I promise. What I would like you to do now is to take a little bit of time and learn how treatments for back pain are proven to really be effective. There are several reasons for you to have this kind of knowledge:

⊙ You will no longer blindly accept a treatment for back pain just because it's offered to you or someone said that it works.

⊙ You won't waste your time and money on ineffective treatments.

⊙ You can get relief from pain as quickly as possible.

By showing you how to tell if a treatment for back pain has been shown to work or not, you will also see that there is good evidence that multifidus strengthening exercises can get results. In addition, you will also become a discriminating consumer of any other back-pain treatments you may come across. Having said that, let's continue.

The Normal Course of Back Pain

The normal course of back pain, or as researchers call it, the natural "history" of back pain, is extremely important to know about for both sufferers of low-back pain and those who treat it. Why? Because we must first know what low-back pain is going to do on its own, without any interfering factors, before we can really say that "x" treatment actually helped it get better. Without such knowledge, we have no idea whether someone's back pain is actually getting better due to the particular treatment that was given, or if it was just the natural tendency of the back pain to get better on its own (Mother Nature, if you will).

It's truly hard to sort out treatment effects without such knowledge. Only when we know the natural tendency of a problem or condition when it is left to continue on its own do we have a yardstick to measure treatments against. As a therapist giving treatments for low-back pain, I am always asking myself if a particular treatment can beat the natural recovery process and change the course favorably. If a treatment cannot, what's the point of wasting the patient's time and money?

Studies on the Natural History of Low-Back Pain

I became very interested in natural history studies early on in my career as a physical therapist as I started treating musculoskeletal problems. I realized then that I needed to know exactly what the natural course of a problem was without any treatment in order to know if I had anything useful to contribute to speed up the natural rate of recovery. When I began my search to locate all the available studies on the natural history of low-back pain, I reviewed more than sixty articles that are supposed to demonstrate its natural course. Unfortunately, I couldn't find a single study on a group of individuals with back pain who were followed for a period of time and had absolutely no treatment at all. A study like this would be the only way to really establish the true course of back pain. So, the next best thing would be to find a group of back patients who had very minimal treatment for their problem, like people who went to the doctor and were given just a medication or prescribed bed rest for a few days.

I was in luck! My review uncovered two studies that had done a pretty decent job of shedding some light on the natural course of low-back pain. The first one was done in 1985 by Gilbert and coworkers and published in the *British Medical Journal*. It took 252 individuals with back pain, with or without pain going into the leg, and no neurological signs present, placing patients randomly into one of four groups. One group got physical therapy, back-education information, and bed rest of at least four days. The second group got physical therapy and back-education information. The third got bed rest (at least four days), and the last was the control group that got none of the above treatments except pain medications—which all the other groups received as well. Patients were followed at roughly ten-day intervals for a month, or until they were pain-free, and again at one year.

Surprisingly, this randomized, controlled trial showed two important things. First, the median time that it took people to return to mild or less pain was two weeks. The second was that all groups recovered at the same rate regardless of which treatment they received. In other words, most people recovered in two weeks, and it didn't matter if they got physical therapy, bed rest, or just pain medications! One year follow-ups showed the same results—no significant differences between treatment groups and everyone having similar levels of pain.

The second study, also in the *British Medical Journal*, was done in 1994 by Coste and coworkers. This time, 103 patients with acute low-back pain not extending below the buttock were studied. No patients had any neurological signs. Patients' pain had to have started less than seventy-two hours before entering the study—an important point when trying to determine back pain's natural course and one that makes this a rare study.

Patients were prescribed only a pain medication and some were put on bed rest or sick leave at the discretion of the doctor. No other treatment was described in the study. Follow-up visits were at day eight, and if the pain lasted, on the fifteenth, thirtieth, and ninetieth day. Once again, a large majority of patients recovered fairly quickly. Pain lasted a median time of seven days, while 90 percent were recovered in just two weeks.

Now let's take the above research mumbo-jumbo and apply it to practical, everyday situations. We have established that back pain improves significantly with only very conservative therapy for most sufferers over the first two weeks of onset. Therefore, wouldn't *any* treatment given to a person during these first two weeks appear to show an improvement? This is very important to know, and I believe it explains why, for example, one therapist uses traction and says it works, while another uses manipulation and says that it works well, too. The truth of the matter is that you could probably have a person stand on their head in a corner as a treatment during the first two weeks of having back pain and it, too, would seem effective. *Anything* will probably appear very effective at treating back pain in these early stages because the majority of people have a tendency to improve *regardless* of which treatment is used. Many seemingly off-the-wall treatments for low-back pain have been concocted without any scientific validation or proof. Natural history explains why proponents of any of them can claim a high rate of success during the initial phases of low-back pain. So keep this in mind the next time you have an acute attack of low-back pain. The chances are good Mother Nature will be doing more for your healing than some fancy new treatment. In fact, advice to continue ordinary activities as normally as possible is supported in multiple, multiple studies as being a very effective treatment for acute low-back pain.

The Randomized, Controlled Trial

So what's a back pain sufferer to do? Dealing with back pain is bad enough without having to get a degree in research to figure out what's really going to help and what isn't. Well, rest easy, because I am going to make it very simple for you tell what treatments have been proven to be effective at fighting low-back pain and which ones are plainly just a hit-or-miss venture.

Anecdotal Evidence

One of weakest types of evidence or proof that something is actually effective is what is known as anecdotal evidence. This is saying that something really works because you tried it and you got a good result. I believe that most good treatments start out this way—trying something and having certain degree of success. However, there are problems with relying solely on this type of proof. Let me show you what I mean with an example.

Let's say that you wake up one morning with a terrible pain in your shoulder. It's nothing you would run to the emergency room for, but nonetheless it hurts. You then remember seeing a commercial on the television the other day that advertised magnets as a way to relieve just about any pain anywhere. "What have I got to lose?" you say to yourself as you walk over to the refrigerator, pluck off a magnet, and tape it to your sore shoulder.

The magnet stays taped to your shoulder all day long, and quite to your liking, the pain is barely noticeable by the end of the day. "Wow," you say to yourself, "these magnets really work!"

A week later, you are shopping at the grocery store and run into a friend. Your friend happens to mention that she has been doing a lot of gardening lately and has some knee pain. Remembering how well the magnet worked on your shoulder, you tell your friend to try a magnet on her knee. This is what is known as *anecdotal* evidence. In other words, the basis for the advice that you gave to your friend to try using magnets on their knee comes from an experience you had—"I tried this once and it really worked!" This kind of scenario is all too common in medicine when it comes to treating musculoskeletal pains. Doctors will say, "I've had patients like you before, and this medication really helped them." Or a physical therapist might say, "I've manipulated the SI joint many times, and it really helps back patients." This kind of thinking is flawed and causes much confusion in the treatment of low-back pain. If we relied just on anecdotal evidence to treat low-back pain, how could we be sure that it was the actual treatment that caused a change, or just a placebo effect? Or, could it have been merely the favorable natural course of the problem? In other words, would the problem get better on its own with time anyway?

Now, the magnet may go on to be the greatest pain reliever of all time, and I did say that most great treatments start out with trying something new and having a degree of success. However, from there a new treatment needs to be properly tested.

In order to assess true treatment effects, researchers have devised something called a randomized, controlled trial. It's the best proof possible to tell if a treatment is causing a real change in a condition, or if the change is merely due to other variables. If a treatment has been shown to work better than a control group or placebo in a randomized, controlled trial, then it has held up to scientific scrutiny. *This is how it will be easy for you to tell if a treatment for back pain has truly been proven to be effective—if it has been demonstrated to be effective in a randomized, controlled trial.* Here's basically how one works.

First you take a group of people you want to treat, let's say people with back pain. Then you pick the treatment you want to test, say magnets. Now we take the group of low-back pain sufferers and we *randomize* them, or arbitrarily assign them to one of two groups—a treatment group that gets to try the magnets out and a control group that gets no treatment at all. This is an important step because when we randomize the back-pain sufferers, we're making sure that no one gets purposely placed in a group that they might do better in (which would influence the results of the study). You can also see that the control group is another, very crucial part of the study. It's what's going to let us know if a person's back pain would have gotten better without wearing any magnets; that is, it "controls" for any other factors involved in a person getting better, such as the placebo effect or the natural history of back pain.

Now that our little trial of magnets and back pain is set up, the next part is to conduct it and then follow-up with the groups over time. Good randomized, controlled trials use objective, valid tools to assess a person's progress during the study. For example, a visual analogue scale like the one below is one such way to objectively measure pain. It's a 100-millimeter line with something like "no pain" at one end and "worst possible pain" on the other. A person can then mark on the line where their level of pain is represented. This makes it easy to compare the pain before the study to the pain after the study, to see if there is truly any change. In this way, it can objectively and accurately be said (and measured) that the pain actually increased or decreased. Most people would probably agree that this is a much better method of showing how well a treatment works than just saying, "People said they felt better after wearing magnets." Things other than pain that could be used to gauge the success or failure of magnets include measuring how far one can bend over or how many activities a person is limited in.

After the trial is over, it's important to know just how long the effects lasted. In other words, as soon as the treatment group stopped wearing the magnets, how long did the decrease of back pain last (assuming of course that the magnets did help with the pain)? This is where follow-up becomes an important issue. A study can be randomized *and* controlled, but if the researchers didn't bother to follow the groups for a period of say, a year, how will we know just how long the effects of the magnets lasted? For example, in our fictitious study, let's say that the magnets were found to make the people who wore them pain-free, and so we concluded that magnets are successful in treating back pain. Hold on a minute. While it may be true that magnets did help people's back pain during the study, we still don't know how long the patients continued to stay better *after* the study was over. What if a few days after the study ended, when people stopped wearing the magnets, everybody's back pain returned to where it was in the first place? On the other hand, what if the back pain never returned and people were eternally pain-free (don't we wish)? We wouldn't have the foggiest clue that any of this happened unless we actually followed up properly after the treatment was finished to see how long the effects lasted. *You can see how just having proof that something worked isn't enough, because it's also crucial to know other things, such as how long the treatment effects actually last.*

no pain ├─────────────────────────────────┤ worst possible
                                                                     pain

date _____

pain site _____

Figure 2.

Those are the essential parts of a well-done randomized, controlled trial. As you can tell, it's much more convincing than the anecdotal evidence described earlier in this section. Unfortunately, it's also a lot more work to do, but I can't think of a better way to really be sure that a treatment is truly effective. When drug companies are testing a new drug, they almost always use the randomized, controlled trial. You probably wouldn't want to use any medication either unless it was properly tested this way, so you shouldn't expect anything less from back-pain therapies. For some reason, medical professionals will often promote a treatment for back pain without first properly demonstrating that it actually works. Television and magazine ads are the worst. I'm not sure why this type of behavior is so commonplace with musculoskeletal problems, with back pain especially falling through the cracks. Health-care professionals involved in treating back pain should rely substantially on evidence from randomized, controlled trials to guide their treatments and get more predictable results. Now *you* know the simple way of finding out if a treatment is effective in relieving low-back pain without getting a degree in research—just find out if there are any randomized, controlled trials that support its effectiveness on your particular type of back pain.

In a Nutshell

⊚ Beware of anecdotal evidence ("I tried it once, and it really works!"). It proves nothing.

◉ Anecdotal evidence does not take into account variables such as the natural course of a disorder, the placebo effect, or any other factors that may influence a good outcome.

◉ Look for randomized, controlled trials done on treatments for low-back pain to tell if they are truly effective or not.

◉ The randomized, controlled trial offers the highest proof of effectiveness that a treatment really works, as it attempts to control for other variables that might influence results.

Randomized, Controlled Trials and the Multifidus

Now that you have been exposed to a little bit of research and have an idea of how treatments are scientifically proven to be effective, it's time to apply this knowledge to the multifidus muscle and back pain.

As I sit and write this book, you need to be aware that there is more and more research coming out all the time about the multifidus muscle. Most of the research that's being done consists of studies demonstrating that there is a problem with the multifidus muscle in people with low-back pain. This is but one of the first steps that needs to be done in order to solve the problem of low-back pain—identifying that there's a problem. And that's exactly what's happening. Researchers are studying different patient populations with low-back pain, such as people with spondylolisthesis, herniated disks, or chronic back pain, and finding out first if problems with the multifidus muscle do indeed exist with these particular types of back problems. The next step, once problems have been consistently and objectively identified, is to take a group of patients with a similar diagnosis, say 100 patients with back pain, identified multifidus dysfunction, and herniated disks, and test a particular treatment.

To date, most of the research about the multifidus has done a fine job of completing this initial step of elucidating the problems that back-pain patients have with this muscle, and these have been discussed in great detail in chapter 2. Research is only now beginning to catch up with the second step, the testing of treatments for multifidus problems. In this section, I'll review randomized, controlled trials that have been done on exercising the multifidus to alleviate back pain. To my knowledge, exercise is the only kind of therapy that has been used so far to help correct multifidus dysfunction in back-pain patients.

The Multifidus, Acute Low-Back Pain, and Recurrences

The first randomized, controlled trial I'll discuss was conducted by Hides and coworkers and came out in 1996 in the journal *Spine*. For those who aren't familiar with this journal (you mean you don't have a subscription to *Spine*?) or don't regularly read back research, it is a peer-reviewed journal that specializes in publishing current back research.

This study took thirty-nine people who were experiencing their first episode of unilateral (one-sided) back pain for fewer than three weeks. No patients had any signs of nerve root compression (such as changes in strength or reflexes). Patients must also have shown a right-left asymmetry of the multifidus muscle (one side smaller than the other) as measured on ultrasound in order to be in the study.

Patients were then randomly placed in a control group or a treatment group (this should sound familiar). The control group got advice on bed rest and absence from work, as well as medications. The treatment group got the same treatment as the control group did, *plus* exercise to strengthen the deep abdominals and multifidus muscles. Pain, disability, range of motion, and the size of the multifidus muscle were then tracked to measure each patient's progress over a ten-week period.

As expected (and keeping with the known course of low-back pain), *both* groups appeared to fully recover by the end of the ten-week study period and were equal in terms of pain, disability, and range of motion. However, what was not the same between the two groups was the size of the multifidus as measured by the ultrasound machine. It was noted that although both groups were feeling and doing much better, the group that did not do multifidus strengthening exercises (the control group) still had an abnormally small multifidus muscle. In stark contrast, the group that did do specific multifidus strengthening exercise had a much more rapid and complete multifidus muscle recovery.

Quite interesting, don't you think? And doesn't this seem to perfectly follow what we know about the natural history of low-back pain? Recall that acute episodes of low-back pain resolve in the overwhelming majority of people in a matter of weeks. However, what I haven't mentioned up until now is that while back pain does go away in a fairly short period of time, it can return over the following year in some 60 to 80 percent of people!

Returning to the above study, it shows us that, practically speaking, you could appear to recover from the low-back pain (as people in the control group did without strengthening their multifidus) and *still* not have normal back muscles. More importantly, this study helps to explain why so many people "recover" from back pain, only to have it turn around and hit them again later some 60 to 80 percent of the time. The pain is gone, but the muscle never totally recovered. Since we know that the multifidus is essential in stabilizing the vertebrae in the back, we can now appreciate how an abnormal multifidus could mean that a person is essentially "set up" for future episodes of back pain.

Let's ponder this theory for a minute. If this is actually the case, then we should see more episodes of back pain over time in the group that still has the puny multifidus muscle, because they did not do the strengthening exercise (they were the control group). And the group that did beef up their multifidus should be doing better over time, being "protected" in a sense from this high rate of returning back pain.

Well, the same researchers continued to follow these patients for a total of three years to investigate if this was indeed going to be the case. Astonishingly, the one-year follow-up revealed that only 30 percent of the group that exercised their multifidus muscles had a recurrence of their low-back pain, which paled in comparison to the nonexercising control group's 84 percent. Furthermore, the three-year follow-up revealed a similar result, with the control group having a 75 percent recurrence of their back pain and the multifidus exercisers a much significantly lower 35 percent recurrence rate. We anxiously await additional studies on this matter for further verification of this phenomenon. However, since reading this research, I have conducted my own "mini" study. I have taken a consecutive series of my patients with subacute low-back pain (for example, the next ten patients who come to see me who have subacute low-back pain) and have given them multifidus strengthening exercises. Then, one to two years after discharging them from therapy, I have one of my students conduct a telephone interview to follow up on them. This interview includes information about pain levels, exercise compliance, and recurrences of low-back pain. To date, everyone that I have been able to follow up with has not had a single recurrence of back pain. Now before we get too excited, remember that my study is small and not a randomized, controlled trial. However, I have also said that great treatments first start out with having a certain degree of success. So for now, let's take these results with a grain of salt. But coupled with good studies like the randomized, controlled trial above, we should also be extremely encouraged that we're headed in the right direction.

What This Study Shows Us

◉ People with acute low-back pain can be demonstrated to have one multifidus smaller than the other on ultrasound imaging.

◉ Acute low-back pain resolves itself in a short period of time.

◉ While pain can get better fairly quickly, this does not necessarily mean that the multifidus is also back to normal.

◉ In short, multifidus recovery is not an automatic thing after the back pain resolves.

◉ The multifidus muscle can be built back up with strengthening exercises.

◉ Future episodes of back pain can be prevented by having a strong multifidus muscle.

The Multifidus and Slipped Vertebrae

The next study I'll discuss was also published in *Spine*, and came out the following year, 1997 (ready to subscribe yet?). This time, O'Sullivan and coworkers decided to test out multifidus-strengthening exercises on a group of patients with either diagnosis of spondylolysis or spondylolisthesis.

As you recall from chapter 2, a spondylolisthesis is when one vertebra slips on top of the other, usually in a forward direction. There are several causes for this, but the one that this study is concerned with is *isthmic spondylolisthesis*. Simply put, this means that the area between the joints in the spine has cracked, allowing the vertebra to slip forward. If the vertebra has a crack in it but has not slipped yet, it's known as *spondylolysis* (pronounced "SPON-duh-LOLL-i-sis"). And that's about as technical as I'll get.

Forty-four patients with chronic low-back pain with or without radiation into the legs participated in the study. Patients also had to have symptoms attributable to the X ray diagnosis of spondylolysis or isthmic spondylolisthesis. Subjects were then randomized to either a specific exercise group or a control group. The specific exercise group trained the deep abdominal muscles and the multifidus. The control group underwent general exercise such as walking or swimming, with a few patients also getting other modalities (heat, massage) and doing trunk curls. Both groups participated in their respective activities for a ten-week period.

Follow-ups were done right after the interventions were concluded and again by postal questionnaire at three, six, and thirty months. Forty-two patients ended up completing the study. Results showed that the group that exercised their deep abdominals and multifidus muscles showed a statistically significant decrease in functional disability and pain. Amazingly, this improvement in both pain and function was maintained, even after the thirty-month follow-up (over two years—fantastic!). On the other hand, the poor control group demonstrated no significant changes after their interventions were completed or even at follow-up.

This is a very strong study with far-reaching implications. Not only was it a randomized, controlled trial, but it had a very long follow-up period of several years. The patients in the study also had somewhat serious back problems—either vertebrae that had cracks between the joints and had the potential to slip or vertebrae that had already slipped. Know that most patients who carry such a diagnosis are usually sent to a surgeon for evaluation of possible surgical stabilization. This usually involves fusing the two vertebrae together, with or without the addition of hardware (such as screws and rods).

Recall from chapter 2 that there are different grades of slips in spondylolisthesis. A grade I is when a vertebra slips 25 percent on the one below it, a grade II is a 50 percent slip, and so on, up to a grade IV. Patients who did have slippage of a vertebra in the study had up to grade II slips. Practically speaking, this means that we now know that strengthening your multifidus can even help people who have at least a slip of 50 percent of one vertebra on the one below it. I don't know about you, but I find this most impressive, especially since it has been demonstrated in a randomized, controlled trial with good long-term follow-up.

What This Study Shows Us

- ◉ Specific training of the muscles that provide stability to the spine can reduce pain and disability in patients with spondylolisthesis or spondylolysis.

- ◉ Surgery is *not* an inevitable consequence when one has a slipped vertebra in the spine.

- ◉ Exercise training involving the multifidus muscle has been demonstrated to significantly help people who have up to a grade II slip (50 percent slip of a vertebra on the one below it)

The Multifidus and Chronic Low-Back Pain Patients

Risch et al. (1993) did a clinical trial that those of us who study back research just love. She took fifty-four patients with chronic low-back pain and randomized them into two groups—a treatment group and a control group. The control group was placed on a waiting list, giving us the ultimate in a control group—subjects that get absolutely no treatment or attention whatsoever, thereby letting their problem improve or deteriorate naturally. And the treatment? Just one specific intervention and nothing more. Patients used a special exercise machine that worked just their low-back muscles in isolation. With this kind of study, one doesn't have to guess exactly what accounted for patients having a change in their pain because there is one, and only one, treatment.

At the end of the ten-week study period both groups were re-assessed. It should come as no surprise that the patients who exercised their low-back muscles had significant increases in back strength. Furthermore, patients reported that their back pain had decreased. In stark contrast, the group on the waiting list reported even higher levels of pain at the end of the study.

What This Study Shows Us

◉ People with chronic low-back pain can make their backs stronger through strengthening exercises despite having long-standing pain.

◉ If a person with chronic low-back pain does nothing more than just a strengthening exercise for their back muscles, they can decrease their back pain.

Other Studies on Exercise and the Multifidus

To my knowledge, these have been the only randomized, controlled trials so far on the multifidus. I find it very encouraging that all of them demonstrated positive results despite the rigors of the controlled trial. There are other studies in the literature involving exercise and the multifidus however, they lack the sophistication of the randomized, controlled trial and are thus less convincing and offer far less proof of efficacy. With the passage of time, though, I'm sure there will be more studies to come that test multifidus-strengthening exercises on different patient populations (such as spinal stenosis or herniated-disk patients, for example), especially in light of the good results thus far.

The rest of the clinical trials that study back problems and multifidus strengthening are mostly nonrandomized and have no control group. Although they show very good results, because of the lack of a control group we have no way of knowing if the patients would have gotten better on their own anyway. The following is a brief synopsis of a few other clinical trials that involve exercising the multifidus.

◉ Lindgren (1993) studied nine patients with vertebrae that moved excessively (as seen on radiography) as people bent forwards and backwards. EMG analysis was also performed on the multifidus muscle, which was also shown to be abnormal. It was noted that the multifidus muscles that were working improperly were, in most cases, at the same level as the vertebrae with the excessive motion. After an exercise program that included stretching, coordination exercises, abdominal- and multifidus-strengthening exercises, the abnormal EMGs practically disappeared. Interestingly though, excessive vertebral motion was *unchanged* at the end of the study, despite eight of the nine patients having painless movement of the spine!

⊙ Rissanen (1995) looked at the effects of training the multifidus in chronic low-back-pain patients. Back-muscle strength was assessed, as well as samples taken of each participant's multifidus muscle. After the participants specifically trained their back muscles (in addition to doing other exercise), researchers found back strength increases of 19 to 22 percent. Also demonstrated was an 11 percent increase in the size of the fast twitch muscle fibers of the multifidus.

⊙ Saal (1989) took sixty-four patients with herniated disks (documented by CT scans) and put them through an aggressive physical rehabilitation program. The key element in the exercise portion was stabilization training, which actively works the multifidus muscle. Ninety percent of subjects had good or excellent outcomes with a 92 percent return-to-work rate. Because other treatments (such as backcare education) were also given to patients, it is hard to sort out treatment effects and say which one helped the most. However, with what is currently known about herniated disks going hand in hand with changes in the multifidus muscle, it's interesting that these researchers showed great results with a program whose key exercise element included working the multifidus.

What These Studies Show Us

⊙ Nothing conclusive at all can be said as far as treatments go, mainly due to the lack of a control group and/or because multifidus training was mixed in with other treatments (how do we know which treatment helped the most?).

⊙ Multifidus muscles can be made to increase in size with exercise.

⊙ Some people with back pain have abnormal electrical activity of their multifidus muscles, as proven by EMGs.

- In many cases, the multifidus muscle just at the level of a vertebra with excessive motion will show abnormal electrical activity.

- Abnormal electrical activity of the multifidus can be corrected with exercise.

Summary

So that's what the scientific studies have to say about back pain and exercising the multifidus muscle. Along the way, I hope you picked up a little knowledge about the natural course of low-back pain. It's actually quite favorable, with acute attacks usually resolving in a matter of weeks for most people. However, back pain does tend to have a high rate of recurrence. Most readers of this book probably suffer from chronic low-back pain and unfortunately have yet to see any long remission periods.

This chapter should be especially encouraging to you. Now is an exciting time for both those who treat back pain and the people who struggle with it, as the research is beginning to now offer practical theories about why some people continue to suffer with back pain. But not only are researchers proposing theories, they are also now beginning to test them in well-done clinical trials. The exercises that follow in the next chapter should be of benefit to most people with back pain, whether it be an acute or chronic condition.

Key Points

◉ The normal course of back pain is quite favorable, with acute attacks resolving within weeks for the majority of people. Only a small percentage will go on to have chronic low-back pain. Back pain tends to have a high rate of recurrence within the first year.

◉ Be wary of using treatments on the basis of, "I tried this once and it really helped," or "I've used this on a few patients like you, and it works great." This is anecdotal evidence and proves nothing as far as a treatment being effective. Anecdotal evidence fails to control for other variables that might really have made the difference.

◉ Look for treatments for your back pain that have been demonstrated to be effective in randomized, controlled trials. This is the highest proof that a treatment really works, as it attempts to control for any factors that might really account for a positive effect.

◉ It has been demonstrated in a randomized, controlled trial that acute low-back pain patients can have a right-left asymmetry of the multifidus muscle, and that doing multifidus and deep abdominal strengthening not only results in a more complete and rapid recovery of the multifidus, but also prevents future back-pain attacks.

◉ Another randomized, controlled trial demonstrated that exercise training involving the multifidus muscle reduced pain and disability in patients with spondylolysis or spondylolisthesis, conditions commonly treated by fusing two vertebrae together with surgery.

◉ It has been demonstrated in a randomized, controlled trial that a person with chronic low-back pain can decrease their back pain just by doing back-strengthening exercises alone.

◉ Other studies have demonstrated that back-pain patients can have smaller than normal multifidus muscles as well as abnormal electrical activity of this muscle, both of which can be corrected through exercise.

4

Getting the Multifidus into Shape—The Exercises That Really Work!

The secret of success is to know something nobody else knows.

—Aristotle Onassis

"So, are you saying that if I exercise my multifidus muscle, all my back pain will go away?" the patient said.

"I never make 100 percent guarantees," I replied. "I haven't gotten my degree in predicting the future yet. But there is a lot of research that has without a doubt shown problems with this muscle in many people with low-back pain. The studies are also showing that you can correct these problems with exercise, so I feel like you'll get at least some benefit from them. They're definitely worth a try."

"Well, what have I got to lose?" said the patient.

"Not much, and besides, doing these exercises won't take much time at all if you use proper strength-training guidelines."

"Really?" the patient said enthusiastically. "The last place I had therapy at had me doing a bunch of exercises. I think I did three sets of ten of each one."

"Yeah, I don't really understand that. It's so well published that if you're just starting an exercise program, one set of an exercise is just as good as two, or even three sets. This has been proven in randomized, controlled trials for quite some time now."

"Well, that's good to know. I'm really not an exercise person."

"Not everybody is. In fact, a lot of people aren't," I said. "But that's okay because you won't have to be a jock to strengthen up those multifidus muscles."

"Sounds good to me. I can't wait to see your exercise program!"

The above conversation is pretty typical of what most people say who come to see me after having had a lot of therapy before. Many patients have been through what I call "the shotgun" approach. No one really knows for sure what the patient's problem is, so the poor patient is hit with a long list of different exercises to cover every possible back problem under the sun in the hope that one of them will work. That's a problem.

Not knowing what's causing a person's back pain is really okay. Actually, the truth is that in the vast majority of cases nobody can *really* tell you exactly what is causing your low-back pain. Over the past decade, I have read literally hundreds of research articles on back pain, in addition to books and many continuing education courses. I now know from all of these experiences that most of the time, *I don't know*. This is a hard thing for a lot of medical professionals to admit. It's like we have failed and let the patients down if we don't come up with the exact cause of everybody's back pain.

To get around the sobering fact that we simply can't pinpoint the exact cause of pain in the majority of patients, while still providing good treatment for people, I have adopted the following strategy. After I have finished evaluating a patient on an initial visit, I place them into two classification systems. The first one has to do with the length of time that the back pain has been present. Recall from chapter 2 the acute, subacute, and chronic pain categories. That's the easy one to place someone in. I use this system because most of the back research has categorized patients this way, and so now I will know which studies and treatments apply to which of my patients. For example, if a person has had back pain less than six weeks, I know to place them in the acute low-back pain group. I can then check out all the randomized, controlled trials that have been shown to be effective with acute low-back pain patients and go from there. Remember that some treatments work better on acute back pain, while others are clearly more effective on chronic.

The next classification system I use also has three groups—serious spinal pathology, nerve-root problems, and mechanical back pain. I credit this system to leading back-researcher Gordon Waddell, a true credit to his profession. For further details on this approach, check out his book, *The Back Pain Revolution* (1998).

Most people, by the time they get to physical therapy, have had serious conditions ruled out by the doctor, which usually takes them out of the first group—serious spinal pathology. These would be conditions such as spinal tumors or infections, for example. Fortunately, this category represents a very small percentage of all back-pain patients. For example, only .7 percent of patients will have a spinal tumor responsible for their symptoms, while an even smaller .01 percent have spinal infections. As you can see, there are some very serious problems for doctors to rule out, but fortunately few people actually have them.

The next group is nerve-root problems, which includes those patients who have compression or irritation of a spinal nerve. If one has any major irritation or compression of a spinal nerve, they should exhibit some of the following symptoms: decreased reflexes in one or both legs, decreased strength in one or both legs, pain in a certain pattern down one or both legs, or changes in bowel or bladder habits. If a spinal nerve is not sufficiently compressed to cause any of these symptoms but is irritated, tests that involve pulling on the irritated nerve might be positive, indicating that this is the case.

Once a spinal nerve is under suspicion as the source of pain, confirmatory tests such as an MRI, CT myelogram, or EMG studies can be done. Of course, these tests should match a person's symptoms in order to be meaningful at all. For example, if a herniated disk is seen on an MRI compressing the L-4 spinal nerve, but the person's symptoms are more consistent with an irritated S-1 nerve, it's probably best then to chalk up the disk herniation seen on the MRI as just an incidental finding. Recall from chapter

2 the high incidence of spinal abnormalities in people with *no pain*. In my experience, it's just not that common to see someone with a compressed spinal nerve seen on an MRI who also has neurological symptoms such as decreased strength, reflexes, or pain patterns that match the same compressed nerve on the MRI. For example, a patient may have symptoms of compression on their L-4 nerve. An MRI is ordered and shows that a disk is actually compressing the L-5 nerve, not the L-4. Like in this example, MRI results seldom seem to match a person's symptoms. In the ten-plus years that I have been treating back pain patients, I have seen only a handful of patients who actually fit neatly into this category. A saying I heard somewhere comes to mind: "If an examiner looks hard enough for something, he will usually see what he or she wants to see." Reliability issues and measurement errors of commonly used diagnostic tests and procedures are also pertinent to this discussion. For example, one might think of radiographs as being a pretty objective piece of evidence to hang a diagnosis on. Each year, for example, many people are diagnosed with degenerative disk disease. One criteria that can be used to diagnose this is by checking a radiograph and measuring the height of the disk that lies between the vertebrae. If the disk is judged "narrowed," this adds to the diagnosis. In reality, one must have a 50 percent reduction of the disk height before they are outside of the potential measuring error—something that must be seriously considered before labeling someone in pain with a "disease." Under a microscope, there is no difference at all between an aging disk and one that has been labeled "diseased." Maybe the bigger question is if aging is a disease. In my opinion, it isn't.

This leaves the last category, mechanical back pain (pain that is generally better when the person is at rest and gets worse with certain motions or positions), which the vast majority of back sufferers fall into. These are persons who have had serious spinal problems ruled out, as well as a negative neurological exam (taking them out of the nerve-root problems group). What's left is to put them in this category.

If you fall into this category, the good news is that there are no serious problems going on in your spine, but the bad news is that I can't really tell you exactly what the problem is. Of course, we can make guesses and theorize, but that's about all we can really do. We just don't have the knowledge and technology yet to exactly pinpoint the true cause in most cases of back pain. Alf

Nachemson, internationally famous back researcher, who is extremely well published, has been quoted as saying, "The cause of low-back pain is unknown in the majority of cases." Being a hard-facts kind of person, I'm with Nachemson. If anyone does know the true causes of back pain in the majority of cases, they need to publish it so the rest of us can be enlightened.

Until then, it has been my approach to categorize someone with back pain into the acute, subacute, or chronic back-pain groups. Then I screen for any signs of serious pathology and rule out nerve-root problems. After these steps have been taken, most people will fall into the mechanical back-pain category. Since I usually don't know what the exact cause of the pain is, I find that the best approach is to treat the function of the back, going on the premise that dysfunction leads to pain—correct the dysfunction, and the pain should improve. This would mean, for example, if your back is tight, therapy is aimed at loosening it up with joint manipulation or stretching exercises. If you have an unstable vertebrae in your back, therapy is aimed at stabilizing it through multifidus-strengthening exercises, and so on. Treating the function of the back bypasses the whole confusing, controversial issue of figuring out exactly what the problem really is when we really can't say so with 100 percent assurance anyway. Here again, I'm not treating a spondylolisthesis (slipped vertebrae) per say, but rather the increased motion (the dysfunction) that is putting tension or compression on tissues which results in pain. Treat the dysfunction (increased motion) and not the diagnosis (spondylolisthesis) is another way of looking at it.

This is exactly what I am attempting to do with the exercises in this book. It's also why I chose this chapter to present the pitfalls of diagnosing low-back pain that you've just read. When you bought this book, you were probably looking for some answers to your back-pain troubles. By this point, some readers if not most will have had certain "labels" placed upon them by the medical community. No longer are you a person suffering from low-back pain, but rather you've become a "degenerative disk disease" patient, a "spinal stenosis" patient, or maybe even a "disk patient" to the medical community. I say let's put down the traditional labels for now and concentrate not so much on treating your given diagnosis, but rather on treating the functioning of your back. I think you'll find that it's a much more logical route to go than trying to treat some questionable diagnosis. I'll jump off my soapbox now and move on to discussing some basic strength-training guidelines from the research. Then we'll move quickly to the part we've all been waiting for—the exercises.

In a Nutshell

◉ Research shows that up to 85 percent of people cannot be given a specific diagnosis concerning their back pain.

◉ There are general categories that back pain can be put into, such as acute, subacute, and chronic low-back pain. Others include serious spinal problems, nerve-root compression/irritation, and mechanical low-back pain. While some categories may not offer specific causes for your back pain, they may be the best description we can confidently offer as far as structural causes go at the present time.

◉ While one can reasonably argue that the multifidus muscle can be a direct or indirect cause of your back pain, this we know for sure: the research clearly shows us that there is a *strong association* between abnormal multifidus muscles and low-back pain and that exercising the multifidus helps. So until we have the adequate knowledge and technology to precisely identify the exact causes and mechanisms of low-back pain, think about treating the *function* of your back and not questionable, traditional diagnoses. This is what multifidus strengthening exercises are really all about.

Facts You Need to Know about Strength Training

The patient in the beginning of this chapter is like a lot of people—she isn't crazy about hefting weights around, despite the fact that it's suppose to be good for her. Well, that's where the good news comes in. If you're one of those people who aren't particularly fond of lifting weights, or exercise for that matter, it's okay. However, this does *not* mean that you are going to get out of exercising altogether (sorry). Despite the fact that you're going to have to do a strengthening exercise to beef up that multifidus, I think that you'll be surprised at how little time and effort it really takes to see results when you use evidence-based guidelines.

A Quick Word about Definitions

Before I begin explaining to you exactly how I want you to exercise your multifidus, I need to be sure that we are all on the same page when using certain terms. The following are some words I will use when discussing multifidus training and what I mean by them.

- *A repetition:* doing an exercise movement one time. For instance, if you are doing sit-ups, bringing your elbows up to your knees and back down again would equal one repetition.

- *A set:* a set is made up of repetitions. A set of ten repetitions of sit-ups would mean bringing your elbows up to your knees and back down again ten times. If you did this only eight times, it would have been one set of eight.

Using the above definitions, three sets of ten sit-ups would mean bringing your elbows to your knees ten times (which is one set) and doing that whole thing three times. Now that we're clear on what means what, let's go over some basic strength-training guidelines.

Research and Strength-Training Guidelines

The first thing one notices when they start reading the strength-training literature in search of the ideal combination of sets and repetitions is one thing—none exists. To put it another way, there is no magic number of sets and repetitions that make up the "perfect" routine. This is true for several reasons. The first one has to do with variety. Let me say now that *any* combination of sets and repetitions that seems to work for you now will grow old, given enough time. Eventually, your rate of improvement will slow, either because you got tired of the same old routine or because your body started adapting to it. The other reason is that different combinations of sets and repetitions have different training effects on the muscles, and because people have different training goals (some need endurance, some strength, and yet others power), no single routine can possibly fit everyone's training needs.

The other thing that makes looking for the best combinations of sets and repetitions so confusing is the fact that you can make strength gains with a lot of different routines. One person might say, "I do three sets of curls and I get good results," but another person will say, "I use five sets of each exercise and it really works!"

While most any routine will result in some strength gains to one degree or another, the research has revealed that some set and repetition schemes do get better results than others. With these ideas in mind, it's probably best to approach the whole thing with the idea that strength gains can be made with a lot of different combinations of sets and repetitions; however, some have been clearly demonstrated in studies to get better results than others. Let's go over repetitions first.

The Lowdown on Reps

Repetitions (or "reps," as you hear people in the gym say) is how many times you do the exercise motion in a given set. Doing any number of repetitions from one to about twenty will result in you getting stronger to some degree or another. However, the piece of information you need to have when weight training is that different numbers of repetitions have totally different training effects on the muscles. The lower numbers of repetitions will train the muscles more for strength (good for tasks such as the quick lifting of objects), while the higher numbers will increase a muscle's endurance more for activities where the muscle must contract repeatedly for a long period of time (such as vacuuming for minutes at a time). Doing repetitions in the middle of one to twenty will give you a mix of both strength and endurance. This is why, if you have ever gone to a gym and started working out, most trainers will suggest a repetition scheme like the classic eight to twelve reps. This repetition set-up gives the muscles a blend of both strength and endurance benefits—two desirable qualities your average person would want. Note that research has shown that anything after about twenty repetitions results in basically *no strength* gains, indicating that the benefits are essentially all endurance at this end of the scale.

Think of the number of repetitions as a continuum. For instance, there is no clear-cut line where ten repetitions are purely for strength only, and eleven is just for endurance. Rather, the qualities combine at certain points, with some numbers distinctively having more of a particular quality than others (such as one being clearly more for strength, and twenty mainly for endurance). Another way to think about this is imagining the repetition numbers sitting on a line. Repetitions that develop strength sit more toward the far left side of the line, and the number of repetitions that develop mainly endurance lie on the right. The following is an example of this.

Repetition number as part of a continuum

1 rep	8–12 reps	20 reps

strength--------------------strength + endurance-----------------endurance

Figure 3.

Sets

Now that you have some idea about what number of repetitions you have to do in order to emphasize training a muscle for strength or endurance, what about the number of sets?

Well, here's where it gets a little hairy. Strength-training programs can be roughly divided into two types, periodized and nonperiodized. Basically, *periodized* programs usually involve doing multiple sets (like around three to five) and changing the repetitions periodically to go from a low intensity to a higher intensity of training over weeks or months. A person then "peaks" at certain times of the year, usually for something like a competition. As you have probably gathered, this kind of a program is used a lot by athletes.

Periodized programs have been found to yield far superior strength gains over nonperiodized programs. So, multiple sets are better than a single set of an exercise if you use them in a periodized fashion. However, it's not necessary by any means to get this involved or sophisticated in order to gain good strength in your multifidus muscle, so this is as far as I'll go with periodization. I mention these concepts only to make sure that you have at least been exposed to all the current research and have all the facts on hand.

In contrast, nonperiodized training programs are the standard type that most people do when they go to the gym and work out. For example, this would be like doing one set of an exercise for eight to twelve repetitions three times a week. Once a person can lift a weight in good form for twelve repetitions, more weight is added. This same set and repetition scheme is done week after week without much change—hence the term "nonperiodized." This is the regimen I would recommend for the average person with back pain who needs multifidus strengthening. Using this nonperiodized training scheme, *one set* of an exercise is all that is necessary to gain satisfactory strength. In fact, studies have been done where one group does one set of an exercise, another group two sets, and yet another does three sets of an exercise. Time and again, the studies on nonperiodized programs have consistently shown that if a person does just one set they get the same benefits as the people who did two or even three sets of the same exercise. The problem is that most of us think that more is better. The truth, however, is that for the average person looking to increase the strength of a muscle, one set is sufficient to stimulate muscle growth, so why do more?

Intensity

Intensity, or how hard you're suppose to push yourself while doing an exercise, is another issue that certainly deserves mention and is a question I am frequently asked by patients. The answer lies in two pieces of information:

1. Doing an exercise until no further repetitions can be done in good form is called *momentary muscular failure*. Research shows that getting to momentary muscular failure or close to it produces the best strength gains.

2. You should not be in pain while exercising.

Taking the above information into consideration, I feel that a person should keep doing an exercise as long as it isn't painful and until no further repetitions can be done in good form within the repetition scheme.

How Many Times a Week?

The last variable we have to discuss is the issue of how many times a week we should do an exercise. Here again, recreational weight lifters and athletes alike have devised many different training programs, all of which will provide a benefit, some more than others. Since I'm writing this book for the average person with back pain whose goal is to exercise their multifidus muscle, I recommend three times a week with a day of rest in between the workout days. Again this is your typical, nonperiodized program shown in multiple studies to increase strength in both the short term and the long term. An example of this would be doing your multifidus strengthening exercises on Monday, Wednesday, and Friday, or Tuesday, Thursday, and Saturday. For that matter, Sunday, Tuesday, and Thursday would work just as well. Just remember the basic guideline—three days a week is optimal, with a day of rest in between workouts. This gives your muscles time to rest, recover, and rebuild for the next workout.

Before I close, I should mention that doing an exercise three times a week is, as I mentioned, *optimal*. But because I'm married, have a full-time job, and two small children, I realize that things do come up for everyone. Life rarely goes by the numbers, and some days we just can't seem to get off the hamster wheel. Fortunately, there has been some good research that tells us that we can also make strength gains by working out only twice a week (I told you exercising your multifidus wasn't going to be that bad).

Yes, as unbelievable as it seems, you can beef up your multifidus (or any other muscle, as far as that goes) by doing an exercise just two times a week. However, there is one little catch. Studies show that while you will gain strength working out twice a week, you will get only about 80 percent of the strength gains that you would have gotten had you worked out three times a week. So, just remember, two times a week doing an exercise is okay, but three times a week is truly what we want to shoot for.

Putting It All Together

It's time for a quick review to make sure you have all the training guidelines down pat. Here's a quick summary of what you need to know about reps, sets, and the frequency of doing the multifidus strengthening exercises.

- ⊚ *Repetitions.* Since the role of the multifidus is primarily that of a stabilizer, it's endurance and a long holding ability that we want to boost the most. I recommend doing either a high number of repetitions (such as twenty), or trying to do an exercise for up to two minutes continuously.

⊙ *Sets.* For your average person with back pain, a non-periodized training program will be good enough to gain all the strength you'll ever need. In light of the current research, I recommend one set of an exercise, once a day.

⊙ *Frequency.* Do an exercise three days a week, separated by a day of rest in between workout days. Two days a week is the absolute bare minimum you can do and still see strength benefits.

What to Expect

That's the nuts and bolts of the strength-training guidelines. On the pages to follow are the exercises that work the multifidus muscle, improving its ability to do its job. As the function of your back gets better, so should your back pain. But what exactly should you expect? Well, everybody is a little different, so I'm a bit reluctant to tell you *exactly* what is going to happen. I can, however, make an educated guess based on experience and research as to how the majority of readers will likely respond.

First of all, you should look for changes in your pain. Sounds silly you say? It's really not. Sometimes my main job is to get a person to see that they are actually making progress and improving. You see, a lot of people come to physical therapy and think that they're going to be pain free right away. If they're still having pain, they start to worry and often become discouraged. The truth is, I have yet to put a patient on a multifidus-strengthening exercise program and have them get instantly better. Better yes, but not *instantly* better. I have found that patients will usually respond to multifidus-strengthening exercises in a quite predictable pattern. One of three things will almost always occur as patients begin to turn the corner and become better:

⊙ Your back pain will be just as bad as always; however, you start to notice it is much less frequent.

or

⊙ You start to notice that the pain is less; however, it is still occurring just as frequently.

or

◉ You start to notice less pain, and it occurs less frequently.

As you notice any of these three things starting to happen, it will be a signal that the exercises are helping. You can then look forward to the pain gradually getting better over the weeks to come. Yes, I did say weeks. Most people whom I have treated, if they are going to benefit from multifidus strengthening, will start to do so after a period of around two weeks. It simply takes this amount of time for a muscle to build up noticeable strength. Then, as the strength of the multifidus steadily increases over time, provided you adhere to the strength-training guidelines in this book, you will build up enough strength in your multifidus to make a difference in the pain you experience. As strength further increases over time, the pain should gradually become less and less. If I dare throw out a rough estimate, three months of consistent multifidus training is usually enough time to see optimal results in pain and function. After that, doing the exercise once a week is sufficient for maintenance.

That's the scenario if the exercises do help your back pain significantly. Being both realistic and having worked with hundreds of back-pain patients, the other scenario is that the multifidus-strengthening exercises fail to help you at all. Unfortunately, some readers may do the exercises exactly as outlined in this book and fall into this category. This should be only an extremely small minority of readers, as most everyone should gain at least a partial benefit from having stronger, fitter back muscles. However, if it is truly the case that you end up gaining absolutely nothing from these exercises, I have included in chapter 6 other treatments that have been demonstrated in randomized, controlled trials to be effective for treating both acute and chronic low-back pain. Hopefully then, no one should read this book and go away empty-handed, as you will at least have a current list of evidenced-based treatments shown to be effective for low-back pain. Sometimes low-back pain can be a multifaceted problem, requiring multitreatment strategies. Strengthening your multifidus may be just one piece of the puzzle and not the whole solution. Either way, you should be off to a good start by toning up your multifidus.

Now that you have a general idea of proper exercise guidelines and what to expect, it's time for the exercises. Don't worry though—I'll be recapping all the exercise guidelines as we go along so you'll know exactly what to do before we're through.

Multifidus-Strengthening Exercises

There are lots of exercises that involve the multifidus and stimulate it to get stronger. But because not everybody has the same back, I can't give you one exercise that will work for every single reader of this book. This is where this process can get kind of hairy, because if you were my patient, I could try different exercises with you and find the ones that work the best for you. Since this isn't possible, I will present a variety of exercises that work the multifidus and leave it up to you and your back to decide which ones you like the best and agree with you the most. **Therefore, I recommend at this point that you continue reading straight through to the end of this chapter to first become somewhat familiar with all the exercises and get a general idea of the body position of each one. Then we'll move on to chapter 5, and I'll discuss actually starting to exercise.** You may be eager to jump in, but remember that your first step is to just get acquainted with the exercises.

Before I begin showing you the exercises, here are a few key rules for you to always keep in mind:

⊙ Always check with your doctor or therapist first before beginning an exercise program.

⊙ The number-one rule is "Do no harm." You should not be in a lot of pain while doing these exercises. Some discomfort is okay—remember that you're working muscles you probably haven't used in a while, at least in this manner.

⊙ Stop the exercise if you have any significant increase in back pain or symptoms. The exercises in this book do not stretch your back significantly or involve any heavy weights and should be safe for your back—however, it's your back and your responsibility to stop if you feel like any harm is being done.

This first series of exercises are my very first choice to give someone for multifidus strengthening. I always have patients try this one initially, as it is done with the low back in a "neutral" or middle position and therefore has the least chance of aggravating anybody's symptoms. In the clinic, it has seemed to agree with about 90 percent of patient's backs.

Multifidus-Strengthening Exercise #1

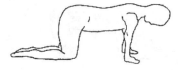

Starting Position

1. You should start on all fours.

2. Your back should be in a middle or "neutral" position (not too bent or too straight, but comfortable above all).

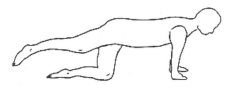

Exercise Movement

1. Raise one leg close to the horizontal, hold for a second, and lower.

2. Try not to let the lower back move while doing the exercise

3. Repeat this sequence with the other leg

4. Do this over and over again, *alternating* the right and left legs, eventually working up to either two minutes or a total of twenty repetitions *with each leg*.

5. Do this exercise one time a day, two to three days a week, with a day of rest in between.

6. When you can do this exercise for either two minutes or a total of twenty repetitions *with each leg*, move on to Exercise #2.

The multifidus muscle can only grow stronger if it is constantly being challenged by some sort of progressive resistance. This is what Exercise #2 does—places a bit more of a load on your multifidus by adding the weight of your arms.

Multifidus-Strengthening Exercise #2

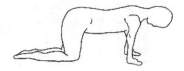

Starting Position

1. Start on all fours.

2. Your back should be in a middle or "neutral" position (not too bent or too straight, but comfortable above all).

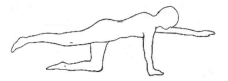

Exercise Movement

1. Raise the right leg and left arm up, close to the horizontal, *at the same time*.

2. Hold for a second, then lower them both.

3. Try not to let the lower back move while doing the exercise.

4. Repeat, except this time raise the left leg and the right arm up, close to the horizontal, at the same time

5. Hold for a second then lower, trying not to let the lower back move.

6. Do this over and over again, *alternating* the right leg/left arm with the left leg/right arm and eventually working up to either two minutes or twenty repetitions (that would be a total of twenty repetitions with the right leg/left arm, and twenty with the left leg/right arm).

7. Do this exercise one time a day, two to three days a week, with a day of rest in between.

8. When you can do this exercise for either two minutes or twenty repetitions (total of twenty times with the right leg/left arm and twenty times with the left leg/right arm), move on to Exercise #3.

This is the last exercise in this series. It's done in exactly the same way as Exercise #2, except this time you are going to add ankle weights to further increase the load on the multifidus muscles. How much weight should you add? Well, that depends. My guess is anywhere from a one- to a five-pound ankle weight on each ankle. I can't tell you exactly because I don't know how much you weigh or how strong you already are. This is where you will have to be the judge. Start out with a pound or two and adjust as necessary so that you are able to do the exercise correctly for at least thirty seconds or so, or if you're counting repetitions, at least ten reps or so.

Multifidus-Strengthening Exercise #3

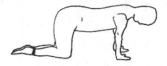

Starting Position

1. Start on all fours with ankle weights on.

2. Your back should be in a middle or "neutral" position (not too bent or too straight, but comfortable above all).

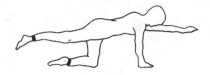

Exercise Movement

1. Raise the right leg and left arm up, close to the horizontal, *at the same time.*

2. Hold them for a second, then lower.

3. Try not to let the lower back move while doing the exercise.

4. Repeat, except this time raise the left leg and the right arm up, close to the horizontal, at the same time.

5. Hold for a second, then lower, trying not to let the lower back move.

6. Do this over and over again, *alternating* the right leg/left arm with the left leg/right arm, and eventually working up to either two minutes or twenty repetitions (that would be a total of twenty repetitions with the right leg/left arm, and twenty with the left leg/right arm).

7. Do this exercise one time a day, two or three days a week, with a day of rest in between.

A Note on Progressing and Maintaining Gains

When you have reached the point where you can do Exercise #3 for either two minutes or twenty repetitions (a total of twenty times with the right leg/left arm, and a total of twenty times with the left leg/right arm) with light ankle weights, you should have built up good strength in your multifidus muscles. Then, to maintain this strength, just do Exercise #3 once or twice a week using the same weight and doing the same amount of time or repetitions as you last did. For example, let's say you feel your back now has good strength and you can do Exercise #3 for two minutes using two-pound ankle weights on each leg. Doing Exercise #3 for two minutes with the two-pound ankle weights on each leg *once a week* is all that is necessary to keep current strength levels. On the other hand, if you feel that your back does need more strength, depending on your goals, job, activities and such, just continue to add more weight to the ankles progressively, a little at a time, until you're where you need to be.

As stated earlier, Exercises #1 through 3 are my number-one choice for strengthening the multifidus muscles. However, there may be a few readers who, for some reason or another, are unable to get on their hands and knees to do the exercises. That's where the next set of exercises comes in. Although they aren't my absolute first choice, they will give the multifidus a workout and succeed in strengthening it nonetheless.

Multifidus-Strengthening Exercise #4

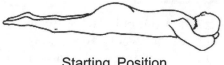

Starting Position

1. Start on your stomach, with or without a pillow under your belly (whichever is more comfortable).

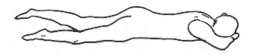

Exercise Movement

1. While keeping your leg *straight*, raise one leg up off the floor, hold it there for a second, then lower.

2. Do not arch your back or lift your leg up too high— around six inches or so is plenty.

3. Repeat with the other leg.

4. Do this over and over again, *alternating* the right and left legs, eventually working up to either two minutes or a total of twenty repetitions *with each leg*.

5. Do this exercise one time a day, two to three days a week, with a day of rest in between.

6. When you can do this exercise for either two minutes or a total of twenty repetitions with each leg, move on to Exercise #5.

Exercise #5 is the same exercise as #4 with the addition of ankle weights to increase the load on the multifidus muscles and challenge it to become stronger. You'll likely need to start out with weights ranging anywhere from one to five pounds on each ankle. Once again, it's hard for me to tell you the exact amount of weight simply because I don't know how big or strong you are. Start out with a pound or two and adjust as necessary so that the exercise can be done in good form for at least thirty seconds or so, or if you're counting repetitions, at least ten reps or so.

Multifidus-Strengthening Exercise #5

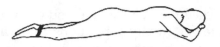

Starting Position

1. Lie on your stomach with your ankle weights on.

2. Place a pillow under your belly, if that's more comfortable.

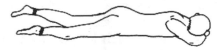

Exercise Movement

1. While keeping your leg *straight*, raise one leg up off the floor, hold it there for a second, then lower.

2. Do not arch your back or lift your leg up too high—around six inches or so is plenty.

3. Repeat with the other leg.

4. Do this over and over again, *alternating* the right and left legs, eventually working up to either two minutes or a total of twenty repetitions *with each leg*.

5. Do this exercise one time a day, two to three days a week, with a day of rest in between.

A Note on Progressing and Maintaining

When you've reached the point where you can do Exercise #5 for either two minutes or twenty repetitions (total of twenty times with the right leg and twenty times with the left leg) with light ankle weights, you are well on your way to building up good strength in your multifidus muscles. To continue to make them stronger, simply keep adding weight to the ankles progressively, a little at a time, until you feel that you're where you need to be, depending on your goals, job, activities, and such. Then, to maintain this strength, just do Exercise #5 once a week using the same weight and doing the same amount of time or repetitions as you last did. For example, let's say you feel that your back now has good strength and can do Exercise #5 for two minutes using five-pound ankle weights on each leg. Doing Exercise #5 for two minutes with the five-pound ankle weights on each leg *once a week* is all that is necessary to keep current strength levels.

So far, I have given you a multifidus-strengthening exercise to be done in the hands and knees position and one that can be done on the stomach. These should cover the majority of readers; however, there still may be someone who can't get into any of these positions comfortably. Maybe you have knee trouble and can't get into the all fours position (or maybe you can, but can't get out of it!). Or maybe your back just talks to you too much while your lying on your stomach. Whatever the case may be, the last exercise will work for you as long as you can either sit or stand. This exercise is known as an *isometric* exercise—that is, an exercise where the muscle contracts but doesn't change its length. It may seem like a puny or trivial exercise, but isometrics have been shown in many studies to be capable of increasing the cross-sectional area (or size) of a muscle on ultrasounds and CT scans. This exercise is a bit tricky to do, so be sure to carefully follow all the instructions carefully. Here is the last exercise.

Multifidus-Strengthening Exercise #6

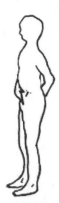

1. Standing is preferable, but the exercise can be done while sitting if needed.

2. Place one hand on your stomach muscles and the other on your lower-back multifidus muscles (see chapter 1 if you've forgotten how to find them).

3. The hands do nothing now, but will feel the muscles tighten later on in the exercise

Starting
Position

1. Tense up your stomach muscles by pulling your belly button in and up while trying to keep your trunk and body still.

2. As you do this, feel with your hands your stomach muscles and your lower-back muscles tense and tighten.

Exercise
Movement

3. Hold this position, muscles tightened, for a count of three to five seconds, and then relax your muscles

4. Repeat, eventually working up to twenty repetitions or contractions in a row.

5. Make sure that when you tense the muscles, you try to do so as tightly as is comfortable.

6. Do this exercise one time a day.

7. Good gains in strength can be made by doing this exercise at least three days a week with a day of rest in between.

8. Doing this exercise daily will bring even better strength gains.

A Note on Progressing and Maintaining

There is no way to add weight to this exercise in order to make it progressively harder on the multifidus. Rather, with isometric exercise, *you* provide the stimulus to keep challenging the muscles by always trying to tense the muscles as tightly as you comfortably can. Continue doing twenty repetitions, holding each repetition for three to five seconds at least three times a week with a day of rest in between, or daily for even better strength gains, until you feel that you're where you need to be depending on your goal, job, activities, etc. For most people, this will probably mean around eight to twelve weeks of consistent exercise. Then, to maintain this strength, just do Exercise #6 once a week. For example, doing one set of twenty repetitions, holding each repetition for three to five seconds once a week while trying to tense the muscles as tightly as is comfortable is all that is needed to keep current strength levels.

Summary

And there you have it, one exercise on the hands and knees, one on your stomach, and one that can be done either sitting or standing. Now that you've been exposed to them all, you'll be able to decide which particular exercise utilizes a position that agrees best with you and your back. Remember though, above all else, *always stop any of the exercises and consult your medical professional if you think any of your symptoms are getting significantly worse*. Once again, it's your back, and your responsibility to take care of it. It's time now to move on to the next chapter, briefly reviewing a few things, tying up any loose ends, and beginning to exercise.

Key Points

⊚ In reality, the exact cause of low-back pain is unknown in the vast majority of cases.

⊚ Rather than trying to treat a questionable diagnosis, think of treating and improving the function of your back instead.

⊚ This is the goal when you do multifidus-strengthening exercises—to improve the functioning of your back.

⊚ Doing a low number of repetitions tends to increase a muscle's strength, while doing a higher number increases mainly muscular endurance.

⊚ Research shows that doing any exercise for over twenty repetitions results in very little additional strength gains. The increased benefits are mainly endurance.

⊚ One set of an exercise is all that is necessary to get good results when one is just starting to strength train.

⊚ With respect to intensity, doing an exercise until no further repetitions are possible produces the best strength gains.

⊚ Doing an exercise three times a week with a day of rest in between each day is optimal, while doing the exercise twice a week is 80 percent as good.

⊚ Look for changes in pain frequency, pain intensity, or both to tell if the multifidus-strengthening exercises are working.

5

Let's Begin

Even if you're on the right track, you'll get run over if you just sit there.

—Will Rogers

"I appreciate all of your help, especially showing me the exercises," the patient said. "I've really learned a lot. Is there anything else I need to know?"

"Probably not," I said. "I think we've covered just about everything you'll need to know to sufficiently strengthen your back muscles. Just remember to stop any of the exercises if they make your symptoms worse. A little bit of discomfort is okay and normal, but most people can tell when something's really wrong. That's when you need to definitely stop. If you start exercising and have any doubts at all, quit and let your doctor know what's going on."

"Okay."

"Now, don't forget, the exercises can't help you if you don't do them. Also, I find that patients are more consistent with their exercises if they pick a certain time of the day that works for them and then stick to that time whenever they do the exercise. For instance, you could do them before you go to bed on Mondays, Wednesdays, and Fridays. Mornings are fine, too."

"That makes sense."

"Give it about three months of consistent exercise to make a firm decision that the exercises didn't do a darn thing for you before throwing in the towel. If you see absolutely no changes at all by then, it's time to switch gears and look at other treatments to try from the list of randomized, controlled trials with your medical professional. One thing I don't like to see is a patient doing the same treatment over and over again if there has been no clear-cut benefit. At that point it's time to move on to something else and stop 'spinning your wheels.'"

"Sounds like a good plan to me," the patient said.

Like the patient I have used as an example throughout this book, you now have all the information you need to start strengthening your multifidus muscles. And if you have fully read every chapter so far, you probably know more about the multifidus and back pain than most patients and a lot of therapists I know. It has taken me a lot of time and patience to dig up and uncover this knowledge, but I am very glad that you've given me an opportunity to share this information with people like you who can use it—that really makes the whole thing worthwhile. I'd like to take a few minutes now to pull together the information you've read up to this point and get you started.

Getting Started

You should be at the point now where you're finally ready to begin exercising. Put on something comfortable—anything that will allow you to freely move your arms and legs will do. If you're doing Exercise #6, the type of clothing you wear makes no difference.

I often get asked if it's okay to do Exercises #1 to 3 on a bed, or whether the surface need be hard. Ultimately, I don't think it really makes that much difference either way. Softer surfaces are definitely easier on the knees, which may benefit some people and allow them to do this exercise. Most mattresses will probably cause your knees to sink down a bit and may even give you added stability, which can make the exercises a tad bit easier. In any case, whether the surface is hard or soft, your multifidus muscles will be contracting and getting a workout.

Picking an Exercise

Start by looking again at the six exercises. Know that *any* exercise you pick from this book will activate the multifidus muscles in your low back. The first series of exercises, Exercises #1 to 3, are my first choice because they strengthen the multifidus muscle in a fashion similar to the way it works in the body. All day long the multifidus is contracting and doing its job as a stabilizer of the spine while we are doing things with our arms and legs—just as in this exercise. Exercises #1 to 3 also challenge the muscle a bit more than the others because you must balance while you do them. This gives the multifidus practice in preparing for situations where you might get caught off balance and be at risk for an injury.

If you can't do Exercises #1 to 3 for whatever reason, don't worry one bit, for Exercises #4 and #5 will also do an excellent job of strengthening the multifidus. The main difference is that Exercises #4 and #5 are not as dynamic as #1 to 3. Nonetheless, I have had many patients who prefer doing multifidus strengthening while lying on their stomachs and still see results.

The last exercise, #6, was put in to make sure that this book had a multifidus-strengthening exercise that everyone would be able to do. It may seem like quite a puny exercise, but if done correctly, it has been confirmed by ultrasound imaging to make the lumbar multifidus muscles bigger over a period of weeks. Not bad!

My point in this section is that they are all good exercises, or I wouldn't have even bothered to put them in the book. Might I also suggest that if you grow bored with, say, Exercises #1 to 3, switch to #6 for a couple weeks. Then go back to Exercises #1 to 3, or try numbers #4 and #5. Variety with training will keep both motivation and results flowing.

Keep the Ball Rolling

Keeping the ball rolling, or progression, is one of my biggest pet peeves, so if you'll let me, I'll vent for just a sentence or two.

As I started out my career writing about low-back pain, I would frequently check out other books on the market, not only to see what was out there, but also to see what my patients were reading and what might be needed. A lot of the books I could find on back pain had a section that showed various exercises that the reader could do to help treat their back pain. What struck me right away was that, while the exercise might be a sound one to prescribe to someone with back pain, the poor reader was not given any guidelines whatsoever as to how they should progress with it over time in order to continue seeing results. For example, an exercise might be to lie on your back, lift one leg up and down slowly, and then repeat with the other leg. "Do ten" a book might say, or "Work up to three sets of twelve." That's okay, but once you've done that, then what? You mean if I can do ten repetitions or three sets of twelve, that's all I'll ever need to strengthen my back?

The fact is (and a well-documented fact at that) for muscles to continually get stronger, they need what is called *progressive resistance*. This is to say that the muscles must constantly be challenged over time in order for them to have a reason to want to get stronger. If a muscle can do ten repetitions of an exercise today, and ten repetitions next week, and ten repetitions next month, what reason does it have to get any stronger? This is, in fact, an example of the efficiency of the human body at work. If a muscle can get the job done with "x" amount of strength, why should the body invest its energy and resources in a bigger and stronger muscle when it's not really necessary? Likewise, if we challenge the muscle over time with more repetitions, more weight, or a different exercise, the body readily responds by growing stronger. It's just that simple.

Having said that, I feel much better. Seriously though, the point of all this is that exercise for people with back pain should follow the same rules as everybody else who's trying to get stronger. Why these principles are largely missing from the books in the back-pain section of the bookstore when one can walk over to the weight-lifting books and find them, I have no idea.

Remember these concepts in order to keep the ball rolling. Make sure that *every* time you do your multifidus-strengthening exercise, whichever one you've chosen, try to complete one more repetition or two than you did last time (or increase the time, if you've chosen to go by time). Then add more weight when you reach the target number (either two minutes or twenty reps with each leg for exercises #1 to 5). If you're doing exercise #6, the idea is to keep trying to tense up the target muscles as tightly as possible.

Progressively challenging the multifidus in this manner and periodically switching exercises is the best way to ensure results over the long run.

What to Look For

Okay. So you've read the book, picked an exercise, are working out religiously, and are on the road to a stronger multifidus. What exactly is going to happen next?

That's difficult to predict exactly for several reasons. For instance, I don't know your medical history and I haven't examined your back. This puts me at something of a disadvantage. But on the other hand, I have given these exercises out to many back patients over the years and have noted several predictable patterns that occur with the majority of people's backs. Therefore, I can tell you with some assurance that one of the following things will probably occur:

- ◎ The exercises don't help at all. This isn't likely to happen, but a possibility nonetheless. In my own practice, I would have to say that this realistically occurs in less than 10 percent of patients. This is because there are few backs that will gain nothing from being stronger. I suggest giving it three months of consistent training before placing yourself in this category. But if this is truly the case, it's still not the time to give up and throw in the towel. My advice is to check out the list I've provided of treatments that have been shown to be effective in treating low-back pain in randomized, controlled trials (see chapter 6) with your medical professional. If you have had low-back pain less than three months, you might want to try treatments under the acute/ subacute category. If you have had low-back pain three months or longer, consider treatments under the chronic pain category.

- ◎ The exercises really work! You would know this because your pain is just as bad as always, but it doesn't bother you nearly as often (frequency is less);

or

your pain is noticeably less, although it is still just as frequent as always (intensity of pain is less);

or

your pain isn't as bad now, and it doesn't bother you nearly as often (intensity of pain and frequency are now less).

So if the exercises really didn't help you out much, consult with your medical professional and check out the list of alternative treatments. This list is based entirely on the research done on randomized, controlled trials. I included these alternatives because, after years of treating low-back pain and working with literally hundreds of patients, I discovered the reality that there is just no one, single treatment that *everyone* is going to respond to.

If the exercises do help you (which is highly likely), expect one of the three scenarios presented above to happen. Look for any decrease in pain, frequency of pain, or both to signal that there's something changing in your low back and the exercises are helping. Some of you are no doubt wondering how long you can expect this to take. Once again, I can only propose a "most likely" time frame, that being around two weeks to start noticing any positive changes. It simply takes this length of time for a muscle to build up a significant amount of strength to be able to change your symptoms. As the strength continues to steadily increase over time, you will begin to accumulate enough strength in your multifidus to make an even bigger difference in your pain. Remember, it probably took some time for your back pain to get to this point, so don't expect it to go away in a day. Be patient and put your energy where it will do you the most good. A little positive thinking can go a long way.

Maintaining the Gains

After a period of consistent exercise, you will have gained good strength in your multifidus muscles. This will also mean that you have improved the overall functioning of your back, which should translate into less pain. You have, in essence, given your back a "tune-up." Two questions usually come up at this point.

⊙ "How long will the effects of the exercises last?"

⊙ "Now that I'm feeling better, how do I keep it that way?"

The effects of the exercise, that is the decrease in the pain and/or frequency of the back pain, should be expected to last as long as the multifidus is in shape and able to do its job (provided of course that your medical condition doesn't change and there are no injuries). If you did stop doing the exercises cold after getting rid of your back pain, there is still a good chance that the multifidus, since it would then be in proper working order, would stay that way. However, I do not recommend testing this out to see if it's really the case. You've already done the hard part, and since it requires little effort to preserve the strength you have worked hard to gain, I see no reason to stop investing in a healthy spine.

To maintain current multifidus strength levels and keep symptoms in check, all one need do is a single multifidus-strengthening exercise a minimum of *one time a week*. Yes, I did say once a week. Research has proven that one set of an exercise done one time a week will preserve strength gains, but only as long as it's done at the same intensity as you did when you stopped exercising to increase strength. For instance, say you were doing Exercise #3 using a two-pound ankle weight and could do it for twenty repetitions with the right leg/left arm and twenty repetitions with the left leg/right arm. Your low- back pain is now much improved, so you really don't need to bump up the weight anymore. It is at this point that you're ready for a maintenance program. This sounds like a big deal, but all it means is that you do whatever you left off with once a week. In keeping with our example, this would mean continuing to do Exercise #3 with a two-pound ankle weight and still doing the twenty repetitions once during the week. The "intensity" of the exercise is therefore being maintained, because you kept the same weight and same number of repetitions. And so, your decrease in symptoms will also be maintained. Note what will not work as well:

⊚ Doing Exercise #3 once every *other* week instead of once a week

or

⊚ Using a one-pound ankle weight instead of the two-pound one

or

⊚ Doing fifteen repetitions instead of twenty

Now, you have to admit, that's not a bad deal at all! Simply follow these guidelines, and you should have no difficulty what-soever maintaining all the hard work you've put into improving the function of your back.

The End?

I remember hearing somewhere that a story doesn't really begin until you're through reading the book. Somehow, that saying seems particularly appropriate to this book.

Now that we've covered the heart of the book (the exercises), and are closing in on the final pages, you probably have more knowledge about your back than you ever did before. And hopefully you have picked up a vital "tool," the multifidus-strengthening exercises, to help relieve your back pain. Use it to help put yourself back in control of your body once again.

They say that the journey of a hundred miles begins with the first step. If that's true, then the steps you've taken thus far in your journey to eliminate your back pain have led you to read this book. It's time to take a few more steps now by giving these exercises a good try using the guidelines provided. When you do, I'll just bet you'll be closer than ever to your destination.

I've dedicated the rest of the book to providing you with many interesting facts about back pain that I often discuss with patients during the course of their physical therapy. Since I can't talk to you personally and don't want you to get left out, I have set up a question and answer format in the next section that will enable you to gain similar benefits as you would if you had been one of my patients. I think you'll find this information extremely enlightening, as this is simply information that never seems to reach the ear of most back-pain sufferers. Good luck, and once again, I have really enjoyed sharing the information in this book with you!

Key Points

◉ The exercises cannot help you unless you do them.

◉ You can do the exercises wearing anything that will allow you to move your arms and legs freely.

◉ The exercises can be done on any surface that is comfortable.

◉ Pick a multifidus-strengthening exercise by the position that best agrees with you and your back—they all activate the multifidus muscles.

◉ To keep progressing and increasing the strength of your multifidus muscles, *try to increase either the amount of time or repetitions each exercise session.*

◉ Switching multifidus-strengthening exercises from time to time is another great way to challenge the multifidus muscles and keep the gains coming.

◉ Look for changes in pain frequency, pain intensity, or both to tell if the exercises are working.

◉ If, after three months of consistently doing the exercises as described in this book, you feel that they have not helped you in the least, get together with your medical professional and check out the list in chapter 6 of treatments for low-back pain shown to be effective in randomized, controlled trials.

◉ After you've reached your goal, doing a multifidus-strengthening exercise once a week at the same intensity you've built up to is all that's necessary to maintain all the benefits acquired.

6

Information *Every* Back-Pain Sufferer Needs to Know

Knowledge rests not upon truth alone, but upon error also.

—Carl G. Jung

"Well, thanks again," the patient said as she started leaving, "I certainly intend to give these exercises a good try. I was wondering though, if there has been all this research done on this muscle, how come no one ever told me about it? I mean I've never been given any exercises like this before, and I've had a lot of physical therapy."

"I wish I had a good answer for you," I replied, "but I don't. My guess is that in a lot of cases, medical professionals don't always keep up with the latest research or regularly read professional journals. It's a shame, but the information I've given you today has been out there for quite some time."

"Really."

"Yeah, it has," I said. "But this kind of ignorance isn't only about information like the multifidus. It extends to other things like the myth that sitting up straight is the best way to sit. If you read the research, you'll see the evidence shows that it's actually good for most backs to sit in a slightly slumped position."

"Hmm," she said.

"Somehow myths like these get started with well-thought-out, logical theories. Eventually though, most end up either having no proof to support them or facing a lot of research showing that they're really not true."

"Well is there any literature you could suggest that can teach me more about back pain?"

"There really isn't any good source I could recommend right now," I said, "other than academic textbooks that probably won't mean much to you. However, I am working on this book about low-back pain . . ."

Unfortunately, the above is true. After reading much literature from peer-reviewed journals over the years, I have come to the realization that there are a lot of misconceptions about back pain out there, as well as plain old myths that haven't a shred of evidence to support them. And that's what this section is all about—to help clear up some of this misinformation so you'll become a much better-educated individual where your back pain is concerned. I'll use a question-answer format to make this section easy to read.

What's the Best Way to Sit?

This is a question I get asked a lot. If you asked me this when I first graduated from physical-therapy school, I would have told you to sit up straight and use a small pillow or towel to support your lower-back curve. However, after reading much orthopedic back literature, I am far from convinced that sitting up straight is the best posture for the spine from a mechanical standpoint. Here's what the literature from peer-reviewed journals has uncovered about the sitting posture. (Please note that terms like sitting "slouched," "slumped," or with the back in a "slightly forward bent position" are all used to mean the same thing—the opposite of sitting up straight.)

1. A radiographic study by Fahrni and coworkers (1965) done on members of certain tribes that live in undeveloped jungle environments and who habitually sit or squat in positions that greatly bend the back show that they have considerably less degenerative changes in the disks than more urban people. One would think that if this bent lower-back position was so horrible and detrimental to your back (the same position that these tribe members spend much of their time in) that they would have the worst looking spines on radiographs. Isn't it interesting that they actually had healthier disks than you or I?

2. There is less stress placed on the facet joints, the small joints of the spine, when one sits in a "slouched" position. This is because sitting up straight actually pushes the two sides of the joint closer together, making them come into more contact with each other. This in turn creates more compression at the joint surfaces.

3. The flow of nutrients to your spine is actually better when you sit in a flexed or "slouched" posture. The better the supply of these vital nutrients, the better off your spine is. I can only speculate, but perhaps this is one reason why the tribe members mentioned above had better disks than other people.

4. *Creep*, that is, the continued deformation of tissues (like the disks) over time in response to a sustained load (as in sitting), is greater when one sits up straight than when sitting slouched. In layman's terms, this means that sitting up straight makes the spine measure shorter after a period of time than when one sits in a slouched position. This is because the tissues are deformed more while sitting straight compared to sitting with the spine bent.

5. Sitting in a slouched or flexed posture dynamically widens and opens up the neural foramens (holes) where the spinal nerves pass through. This can be especially beneficial in conditions such as spinal stenosis, where changes brought with increased age narrow these holes, thus creating the potential for nerve compression. On the other hand, sitting up straight makes the spine move into backward bending, which makes these holes smaller.

And now the evidence for sitting up straight:

1. Sitting up straight increases disk pressure. This is true, but it has never been shown that this is a bad thing for a normal back. Incidentally, every time you contract your muscles, the intramuscular pressure (pressure inside the muscle) also shoots up as well. Increased pressure is just part of the way things work in our bodies as we move. Furthermore, in the sitting posture, the compressive force of the spine is about 1000 newtons, or less than one-tenth of the force required to actually cause failure of the spine.

2. Your mother probably told you to.

All jokes aside, my point is that there is really no conclusive evidence in peer-reviewed journals that pinpoints sitting up straight as being the optimal posture for your back. In fact, the evidence appears to point in the opposite direction—sitting in a flexed or slouched position. Now that you have the above knowledge at hand, I'll tell you my answer to the question, "What is the best way to sit?" It is threefold.

- ◎ From a mechanical standpoint, the best way to sit appears to be with the back in a slightly flexed or "slouched" position. Let's face it, it's a position we all seem to end up in anyway.

- ◎ Of course there are always exceptions to every rule. An obvious example is a patient with a confirmed acute disk herniation. For instance, let's say that you bent over to lift a heavy box, perhaps felt a "pop," and an MRI shows a herniated disk that exactly matches your symptoms. In this case, I would advise sitting up straight with a support for your lower back, at least until symptoms improve. We do know that sitting slumped and with the back in a flexed position does indeed increase disk pressure—something obviously not good for an acute disk herniation that's trying to heal. But then again, I have never met a patient with an acute disk herniation who was able to sit slouched anyway—it simply hurts too much. Mother Nature seems to know best.

- ◎ My bottom-line answer—sit in the position you are most comfortable in and stop feeling guilty for it!

Can Manipulation Restore a Vertebra That's Out of Place?

My first instinct is to offer you my condolences, because in order for you to actually have a vertebra out of place means that you've probably sustained some kind of severe trauma, like getting hit by a car or falling from a tree. It's unlikely that your average person doing average activities is going to have one of their vertebrae suddenly become displaced without some kind of forceful event having taken place.

Patients confronted with a medical professional who claims to have found a vertebra out of alignment and purports to be able to put it back in place needs to ask two questions. One, how did the vertebra get out alignment in the first place, and two, what's going to keep it there once it's put back?

This is an issue I was confronted with early on when I first started to specialize in back problems. I did then what I still do to this day when I come across controversial issues—fall back on the research to help resolve them. Here are some pertinent findings from my own literature search on manipulation and "out of place" vertebrae:

1. First of all, positional faults, or vertebrae falling out of normal alignment, have yet to be scientifically demonstrated to actually exist.

2. Secondly, even if minor displacements of the vertebrae did exist, the possibility of someone being able to find them manually is quite low. Most practitioners (such as chiropractors), use techniques with their hands to determine which vertebrae are the ones that are out of place. The literature is very consistent when it comes to the reliability of manual techniques—most all have extremely poor intertester (between testers) reliability. This means, for example, that two chiropractors would have a hard time agreeing with each other on which vertebra is the one that is out of place. Reliability has been shown to be equally poor even when it comes to much bigger things, such as two examiners trying to agree on which hip is higher, much less tiny positional changes of the vertebrae.

3. Even if we ignore all of the above facts and assume that, one, positional faults do exist, and two, they can be

reliably detected, it has been scientifically documented that manipulation cannot change the position of vertebrae. In 1978, a study by Roberts and coworkers was published in *Rheumatology and Rehabilitation* where X rays were taken of low-back-pain patient's lumbar spines before and after manipulation. The researchers then objectively measured the positions and angles of the vertebrae in the low back from the spinal X rays. They found no differences between the before and after measurements, showing that in fact no change in vertebral position had taken place with the manipulation.

As you can see, no solid evidence exists that you can actually have a vertebra out of alignment, short of a traumatic episode. Even if you do accept that vertebrae do get "out of place," conclusive evidence from X ray studies show that manipulation cannot alter the positions of the vertebrae anyway. Medical practitioners who use unreliable manual techniques to diagnose malaligned vertebrae, a condition that has never been scientifically demonstrated to exist, and then claim that they can return them to their correct position have surely missed the mark.

Is Manipulation Useful at All in Treating Low-Back Pain?

Absolutely! In fact, it has been shown in *multiple* randomized, controlled trials to be effective with acute low-back pain and works even better with chronic back pain patients. After reading the answer to the last question, you're probably looking a bit puzzled at the moment, so let me explain. I do not use manipulation because I believe that I'm actually putting vertebrae back in place; rather, I use it to loosen up tight joints in the spine. Here's my rationale for the use of manipulation with back pain:

1. Manipulation has been shown to be effective in treating both acute and chronic low-back pain. It has passed the rigors of the randomized, controlled trials described in chapter 3.

2. It has been demonstrated that manipulation is incapable of putting vertebrae back into place, so when I do use it to treat low-back pain, it's not with that purpose in mind.

3. Manipulation has been shown in studies to increase the range of motion of a joint. I therefore use manipulation to free up any tight joints patients might have in their spine. These would be the facet joints that help link the vertebrae together.

4. I stated earlier that reliability using manual diagnostic techniques is generally very poor. There is a technique that I use that has demonstrated good intratester reliability (can you get the same result consistently if you went back and tested it again) but still has poor intertester reliability (whether two examiners agree on the same finding). I therefore couple my findings from the hands-on technique with an objective tape-measure method to ultimately decide if your back has any tight joints.

5. All of this assumes that there can indeed be tight joints in the spine. These joints, the facet joints I have mentioned here and there throughout this book, are "synovial joints" just like most of the other joints in your body, such as the knee or the shoulder. One characteristic of a synovial joint is that it has a joint capsule. This is tissue that encloses the joint and has been demonstrated in studies as having the ability to become tight and restrict joint motion. A common example you may have heard of is "frozen shoulder." This occurs when the shoulder capsule has tightened down around the shoulder joint rendering a person incapable of moving their shoulder very much at all. Another example is a broken arm newly coming out of a cast—elbow motion is limited due to both a shortened muscle and a tight joint capsule because the arm has been immobilized for an extended period of time. The facet joints in the spine act no differently—they, too, can become tight. Decreased motion then should be the primary reason for manipulating a spine.

As you can see, manipulation is a quite useful tool when it comes to treating low-back problems. However, you must realize what's actually taking place when one manipulates the spine. I tend to treat the joints in the back just as I would any other joint in the body, just as I would your knee, for example. I simply do not have any research to tell me to do otherwise.

Furthermore, I have found that evaluating the motion of each vertebral segment in the spine is one of the most frequently overlooked items in spine evaluations. If someone seeks medical attention for, say, shoulder pain, the range of motion in that shoulder is almost always checked. Not only would a medical professional see how high *you* could lift your arm up (this being your active range of motion), but the examiner would also take your arm and see how high *he or she* could raise it as well (this being your passive range of motion). For some reason, this same thinking doesn't seem to be applied to the spine, with passive vertebral motion usually overlooked.

As for the "pop" that is frequently heard with spinal manipulation, that's merely the release of a gas bubble in the joint. A vacuum is created when one "gaps" the joint during the maneuver, causing the gas to "pop" out. Sorry, nothing as dramatic as putting one's vertebrae back into position going on here.

How Long Should I Hold a Stretch?

First know that stretching used in isolation (by itself) has not been proven in randomized, controlled trials as an effective treatment for low-back pain. So I can't recommend stretching as a stand-alone treatment for your back pain. Having said that, I feel that there are two reasons to stretch. They are:

◉ To increase the length of a muscle

◉ To relieve muscle tension

The stretching guidelines are distinctively different for each, so before you stretch, first decide exactly *why* you are stretching. If you're stretching to relieve muscle tension, then a few seconds of stretching is all that is necessary. Examples would be if you got a sudden cramp in your calf muscle or had been typing at your computer for a long time and your neck muscles became tense from being in one position. A few seconds of quick stretching usually does the job to relieve that tension.

On the other hand, if your goal is to stretch a muscle in hopes of eventually making a permanent length change—say you have tight hamstrings and want to increase your range of motion (to become more flexible)—then the guidelines are a little different.

It has always amazed me that as long as the medical community has been advocating stretching for the body as a treatment, it wasn't until 1994 that a randomized, controlled trial was conducted to demonstrate the optimal length of time and frequency a person has to stretch in order to get the best results. Bandy and Irion conducted two studies, one published in 1994, and a follow-up study in 1997, in the journal *Physical Therapy.* Here's what they concluded from their randomized, controlled trials:

1. In the first study, the researchers focused on four groups. One group didn't stretch (the control group), one held a stretch for fifteen seconds, another for thirty seconds, and the last group for sixty seconds. Each group that stretched did one repetition of a stretch, once a day, five days a week, for six weeks. Results showed that fifteen seconds of stretching was no more effective than no stretching at all. Furthermore, there were no significant differences in the range of motion gained between individuals who stretched for thirty or sixty seconds, showing that thirty seconds of stretching is just as effective as sixty seconds. Taken as a whole, this well-done, randomized, controlled trial shows that stretching a muscle for thirty seconds, one time a day, five days a week is sufficient to stretch out a tight muscle.

2. Their next study went on to try to determine the optimal number of times a day that would produce the best gains in a muscle's range of motion. This again was a randomized, controlled trial, but this time the researchers used five groups. The first group did three one-minute stretches. The second group did three thirty-second stretches. The third did one one-minute stretch, and the fourth did one thirty-second stretch. The last group was a control group and didn't stretch. All the groups that stretched did so for five days a week, for six weeks. Surprisingly, no differences in range of motion were found among any of the groups that stretched. In other words, a person who did one thirty-second stretch, one time a day, gained just as much range of motion as the person who stretched three times a day and held the stretch for sixty seconds!

Based on these two randomized, controlled studies, my current recommendation if your goal is to increase the length of a muscle is to stretch one time a day, hold the stretch for thirty seconds, and do this five days a week. This recommendation does not apply to muscles that have become shortened or severely contracted due to immobility such as being in a cast or on bedrest for a prolonged period of time. Severe muscle contractures such as these require a low-load, prolonged stretch (holding a position for an extended period, say twenty minutes, with a small force applied, such as a weight).

If anyone recommends any different guidelines for static (held still) stretching, you should request that they show you a randomized, controlled trial to support what they say. As you can see, stretching out tight muscles need not be an all-day affair if done properly using evidence-based guidelines.

What Else Can I Do for My Back Pain?

This is a good issue to address as I do not want to mislead readers of this book into thinking that the only and best thing you can do for your low-back pain are multifidus-strengthening exercises. I chose to write this book with the intent of giving back-pain sufferers yet another treatment option that had scientific support and randomized, controlled trials that back up their use. Multifidus strengthening is, however, just one of a variety of treatments that have evidence of effectiveness against low-back pain and just one tool I have in my toolbox to use with patients.

At regular intervals, I scour the current literature to keep up with the latest findings of what has been shown to be effective in treating low-back pain. The current list that I'm providing for you comes from my own synthesis of two sources. The first is a study that was published in *Spine* in 1997. Van Tulder, et al., took the enormous task of compiling all the randomized, controlled trials of common treatments for low-back pain from huge databases from the years 1966 to September 1995. Not only did they compile all the randomized, controlled trials, but they rated them on their methodological quality, to boot—remember that not all randomized, controlled trials are the same (for example, some might have a longer follow-up period, which makes it a better study).

Several years after the above article was published, an academic textbook, *Neck and Back Pain: The Scientific Evidence of Causes, Diagnosis, and Treatment* (Nachemson 2000), came out. It was published mainly for medical professionals who treat back and neck pain. It includes several chapters that list the effectiveness of treatments for acute, subacute, and chronic back pain according to randomized, controlled trials. I then compared the two sources and created a synthesis of the results. Some treatments were found to have more evidence for being effective than others, and as such, I have listed them below by these different levels of evidence. If any of these treatments do interest you, discuss them with your medical professional.

Effectiveness of Some Treatments for Nonspecific, Acute/Subacute Low-Back Pain

The following information applies to people with non-specific low-back pain (no certain cause identified such as a herniated disk or compression fracture), who have had low-back pain less than three months.

Strong Evidence Found for Being Effective

- ◉ NSAIDS (nonsteroidal anti-inflammatory drugs)

- ◉ Muscle relaxants

- ◉ Advice to continue ordinary activity as normally as possible

Some Evidence Found for Being Effective

- ◉ Epidural steroid injections (only for people with both acute low-back pain **plus** nerve-root pain)

- ◉ Manipulation

- ◉ Traction

- ◉ Behavioral therapy

Contradictory Results of Effectiveness Found Between Studies

- ◉ TENS units

- ◉ Back school

Effectiveness of Some Treatments for Nonspecific Chronic Low-Back Pain

The next list of treatments apply to people with chronic low back pain (pain lasting at least three months or longer) that is of a non-specific nature (no certain cause identified such as a herniated disk or compression fracture of the spine). Once again, discuss any of these treatments that interest you with your medical professional.

Strong Evidence Found for Being Effective

◎ Manipulation

◎ Multidisciplinary pain treatment program

◎ Exercise therapy (no evidence found favoring one particular kind of exercise)

Some Evidence Found for Being Effective

◎ Muscle relaxants

◎ NSAIDS (nonsteroidal anti-inflammatory drugs)

◎ Lumbar corset with a support

◎ Behavioral therapy

◎ Back school

Contradictory Results of Effectiveness Found Between Studies

◎ TENS units

◎ Acupuncture

◎ Epidural steroid injections (for patients with radicular symptoms only)

As you may have noted, the above is not a comprehensive list of every treatment there is for low-back pain, just the more commonly used ones that have been researched the most. Keep in mind also that some treatments, such as magnet therapy, don't have any randomized, controlled trials published yet in peer-reviewed journals to support their effectiveness. It doesn't necessarily mean, just because a randomized, controlled trial hasn't been done yet, that a therapy isn't effective. It merely means that it hasn't been studied enough and we have no proof one way or the other of its effectiveness as a treatment. Remember, too, that each year brings new studies and evidence to further strengthen or refute treatments, so think of the lists I've presented as being changeable, since they are continuously being updated and added to. However, the current lists do represent several decades of research.

A few readers may be puzzled as to why exercise is not included in the list of treatments for acute and subacute, nonspecific low-back pain. This is because no exercise, even multifidus-strengthening exercises, have been demonstrated to get people in the acute/subacute stages out of pain any faster than a control group that has minimal or no treatment. This of course makes perfect sense when one considers the natural course of low-back pain. Recall the randomized, controlled trial presented in chapter 3 dealing with patients with acute back pain. Both groups of patients got better whether they had worked on strengthening their multifidus or not. Indeed, Mother Nature seems to be the best healer of all, at least in the acute stages of low-back pain. I do, however, strongly advocate acute low-back pain sufferers doing multifidus-strengthening exercises, not to get out of pain faster, but to prevent recurrences.

You will also notice that in the list of treatments for chronic, nonspecific low-back pain, no evidence has been found favoring one particular type of exercise over another. This is simply due to the fact that not enough randomized, controlled trials have been done yet with multifidus-strengthening exercises and this specific patient population (chronic-pain patients with nonspecific low-back pain) to draw firm conclusions. Here again, I still highly recommend multifidus strengthening for most chronic-pain patients for three reasons. First, the evidence clearly shows that chronic-pain patients have distinct problems with their multifidus muscles. Second, studies have also proven that these changes in the multifidus muscle can be corrected with exercise. Third, we do have a well-done, randomized, controlled trial demonstrating that multifidus strengthening can actually decrease chronic low-back pain. Only time and multiple, well-done studies will eventually prove their full efficacy.

Can Multifidus-Strengthening Exercises Help Osteoporosis?

To my knowledge there have been no specific studies that have taken individuals with documented osteoporosis, strengthened their multifidus muscles, and rechecked the status of their bone density after a sufficient period of time in order to accurately assess the effects, and then compared the results to a control group. This is what would have to happen in order to prove that specific strengthening of the multifidus muscle actually helps patients with osteoporosis. But don't get disappointed just yet. Although I seem to be painting a dismal picture, let me tell you what I do know about exercise and osteoporosis, and why I highly recommend multifidus-strengthening exercises to patients with osteoporosis of the spine after their doctor's approval.

For years I recommended walking as one of the treatments to help my patients with their osteoporosis. My thinking, and that of a lot of other people, was that walking was a weight-bearing activity that provided a stimulus to keep the bones strong. Then one day, after reading a very interesting article that questioned the ability of walking to increase bone mineral density in the spine (the denser the bone, the stronger it is), I decided to conduct my own literature review on the subject. Here's what my search revealed:

- Studies show that walking *does not* consistently stimulate bone mineralization in the spine.

- It's far from being clear-cut in the literature that walking is beneficial for enhancing bone mineralization.

- In stark contrast, I found extensive documentation showing conclusively that strengthening exercises *do* increase the bone mineral density in the spine.

- The effects of strengthening exercises on increasing bone mineral density are *site specific*. In other words, the muscles that are working during the exercise are attached to bones. Only those bones that the muscle is attached to and pulls on during the resistive exercise are the ones that are stimulated to increase their bone mineral density. Practically speaking, this means that doing arm curls with a dumbbell might increase the bone mineral density in your arm bones, but will do nothing for your leg bones.

Sounding better all the time, isn't it? Nope, there are no studies yet that have been done using the specific multifidus-strengthening exercises in this book. However, the literature is quite conclusive in regards to strengthening (or resistive) exercises offering site-specific increases in bone mineral density for the bones to which they attach. Since Exercises 1 through 5 in chapter 4 utilize progressive resistance with the use of weights *and* contract muscles that attach directly to the lumbar vertebrae, I feel confident that they are very beneficial for an osteoporotic lumbar spine and recommend them to patients after they have been given the go-ahead from their doctor.

Will Losing Weight Help My Back Pain?

In my opinion, blaming someone's low-back pain primarily on their weight is usually just an act of scapegoating when an examiner has failed to find any other reasonable explanation that can account for the pain. I admit it's tempting and even logical. Patients also bring it to my attention at times, saying something like, "Do you think my weight has anything to do with it?" My reply used to be, "Well, it's possible. Certainly losing some weight couldn't hurt." That's what I *used* to say.

In 2000, an article by Leboeuf-Yde came out in *Spine* that discussed the available literature and what the bottom line is regarding the link between back pain and body weight. This was by far the most comprehensive review on the subject I have ever read, and I still haven't found another analysis that has done as good a job. Here's a brief synopsis:

- ◉ Reviewed in this study were some sixty-five articles on weight and back pain.

- ◉ Sixty-eight percent of the sixty-five studies showed no association between obesity and back pain.

- ◉ The author concluded that after about thirty years of research on this topic, there was not enough evidence to determine that body weight is a true cause of low-back pain.

So, contrary to popular belief, the majority of studies actually show no link at all between being overweight and having low-back pain. Additionally, I do not know of any evidence showing that losing weight is effective for treating low-back pain.

Now, I am very much in favor of a person losing their excess pounds, but for general health reasons—not as a specific treatment for back pain. If you are overweight and suffer with low-back pain, I would investigate reasons other than your weight as the primary cause of your problem.

Am I Doomed?

"If I've been diagnosed through X ray and MRI with terrible degenerative changes I can't even pronounce, am I doomed to have back pain for the rest of my life?"

You absolutely are not doomed to a life of back-pain misery. What you can expect, however, is the occasional back pain that the rest of us have. I much prefer to call what was seen on your imaging tests as the expected changes with age that we all are "doomed" to get, provided we live long enough. Welcome to the human race—you're in good company.

I've been working in a hospital for many years now, and when I'm not busy treating outpatients with back pain, I'm up on the floors providing physical therapy for the inpatients. Over the years, I have treated patients with just about any disease you can name. One thing I have learned is that the human body is just not made to last forever. However, at risk of getting into a theological discussion, I really can't believe that our destiny is to be condemned to a life of pain as our body wears down with normal wear and tear over time. While the human body isn't perfect, it's certainly made better than that and in my travels I have seen it withstand more disease than I ever thought it was capable of taking. Let me go over what aging changes a *pain-free* spine can happily live with to lend a little support to my views and help demonstrate my point. Here are a few facts from a literature search I did on abnormal findings in pain-free individuals:

- ⊚ It is well documented that the disks in your spine normally start showing aging changes when you are in your early twenties. Yes, I did say twenties. This has been shown to be true in both cadaver studies and studies on living people with no back pain.

- Bet you didn't know that disk "degeneration" can also be found in children. The journal *Radiology* published a study in 1991 by Tertti and coworkers that compared the spines of thirty-nine fifteen-year-old children with *no* back pain to thirty-nine fifteen-year-old children *with* low-back pain. MRI scans showed disk "degeneration" present in 38 percent of the children with back pain and in 26 percent of the fifteen-year-olds with no back pain. This means over a quarter of fifteen-year-olds can show disk "degeneration" and still not complain of any pain. I'm sure that if someone told those fifteen-year-olds with no back pain that they had disks that were "degenerating," they would probably begin to think much differently about their backs and have a better chance of complaining of back pain down the road.

- There is no difference anatomically between an aging disk and a disk that has been said to suffer from "degenerative disk disease."

- There is no firmly established relationship between low-back pain and what is called "disk disease."

- It's interesting to note from the epidemiological back literature that the peak prevalence of low-back pain is between the ages of thirty-five and fifty-five. If one assumes that "degenerative" changes such as spinal stenosis or degenerated disks are major causes of low-back pain, then why does back pain rear its ugly head mostly in midlife as opposed to when people are older and clearly have more "degenerative" changes? This just doesn't add up.

- You can have pressure on a spinal nerve root (caused by a disk, for example) and have no pain whatsoever. A normal nerve that is compressed will not produce pain. The nerve has to be irritated or inflamed first.

- Abnormalities such as compressed nerves, herniated disks, bulging disks, Schmorl's nodes, spinal stenosis, and facet-joint degeneration have all been found to exist in people with no low-back pain in numerous studies.

I could continue with many more interesting facts, but I think you can see what I'm getting at. Now you know why I'm usually not impressed by most findings of structural changes to the back unless they correlate extremely well with a person's symptoms. I have found that this usually isn't the case with most back problems if one goes into a back evaluation with an open mind and relies on as much objective evidence as possible. One must also remember the limitation of tests used to diagnose back problems and consider factors such as reliability, specificity, and sensitivity. Take all these things into consideration and it's really not that often that I can truly correlate many patients' symptoms with a structural finding seen on an imaging test.

While we're on the subject of normal "abnormal" findings, let me say that this is yet another reason that treating the multifidus muscle has made sense to me. You just don't have all these studies in the literature showing abnormalities with the multifidus muscle in people with no back pain, in contrast to all the other degenerative changes mentioned above. Problems with the multifidus do indeed seem to stand out in people with back pain but are hard to find consistently and to any great degree in pain-free individuals.

Of course, there are cases where aging changes in the spine can be responsible for a person's back pain. And we now know that these changes occur in a quite predictable manner that is well documented in the literature. The course of events that produce "degenerative" or aging changes in the spine occur in three distinct stages:

- ◉ *The dysfunction stage.* The current thinking suggests that problems start in the disk first as a result of minor (or major) mechanical trauma. Examples would be a tear or bulge in the disk from perhaps an auto accident or heavy lift.

- ◉ *The instability stage.* Mechanical trauma to the disk can make it "thinner," which in turn makes the vertebrae it sits between come closer together. As the vertebrae come closer together, this action stretches the joints. The net effect of this results in increased motion and the vertebrae becoming more mobile. And this mobility causes further changes to occur in the disks, vertebrae, and joints as the spine tries to stabilize itself. It is at this point that one see things such as osteophytes (bony overgrowths) or enlarged joints. Sometimes these changes can crowd out spinal nerves and create symptoms.

⊙ *The stabilization stage.* The spine continues trying to stabilize itself until these changes (such as the enlarged joints or extra bone laid down) have successfully decreased motion of the vertebrae. It is then that the spine has reached the stabilization stage.

As you can see, problems start with some sort of trauma to the spine, particularly the disk, which in turn produces other changes that eventually cause increased motion of the vertebrae. Given enough time, the spine will seek to stabilize itself and succeed in doing so. This is usually not until a person is much older, though. It's these attempts that the body makes to stabilize itself and decrease excessive motion that end up crowding the spinal nerves out. This is one reason why I feel that multifidus strengthening becomes so important in patients who have any kind of instability or aging changes (like spondylolisthesis or spinal stenosis). Ligaments, which connect bones to bones, lose their ability to adequately hold the vertebrae together. This is part of the "passive" system that the spine has to stabilize itself. So if that system is failing, we can fill the need by beefing up the "active" system with strong multifidus muscles. Needless to say, I am anxiously awaiting randomized, controlled trials to prove this an effective treatment in patient populations with conditions such as spinal stenosis.

Before I close this discussion, let me note again that pressure on a spinal nerve is not enough to cause pain. The nerve has to be irritated or inflamed first before any pain occurs. In other words, a spinal nerve *with* irritation and inflammation will be sensitive to aging changes, such as bone spurs, and cause pain. Normal spinal nerves that are not irritated and free of inflammation will not be sensitive to the bony spur compressing it. It's truly amazing what a spinal nerve can take while still not producing any symptoms.

A practical application of this knowledge could be a case where an elderly person with no prior history of back pain gets into a car accident. The person has sustained no serious injury during the accident, but is left with terrible low-back pain and pain also going down into the leg. Reflexes are found to be decreased in that same leg. Eventually the person is referred to a surgeon who takes X rays and MRIs. The results show severe aging changes in the low back. A myelogram is then done and shows a compressed spinal nerve. Surgery is recommended.

What would you do if this were you? Would you have surgery? I mean after all, this is a spine with severe aging changes and a compressed spinal nerve for crying out loud!

Maybe not. Let's take some of the facts we've learned thus far and apply them to this case. First of all, this is an elderly person who had no pain before the car accident and lived just fine with their aging changes. There may have been some spinal-nerve compression, but since the nerves weren't irritated, they caused no problems. This makes sense and has been well demonstrated in studies on people with no back pain. Therefore, since we know the person can live with these aging changes quite well, having surgery to take pressure off the nerves with surgery may not be the only option.

Now, it's true that the cause of the back and leg pain could be from an irritated spinal nerve, especially because the patient has neurological signs (the decreased reflexes). If this is the case, the spinal nerve is most likely inflamed and irritated from trauma (the car accident), and all those aging changes that the person lived in harmony with before *now* become an issue and cause problems. They are perpetuating factors, if you will. In other words, since the nerve is now inflamed and irritated, this makes it sensitive to the pressure from the aging changes it lived with before. The key, therefore, is not to cut out all the bony spurs and such, but to get the irritation and inflammation down. Once this is accomplished, the nerve can go back to coexisting with all the aging changes quite nicely again. Just remember, normal nerves don't cause pain when pressed on, but nerves that are irritated and inflamed do. This is one reason why epidural steroid injections have proved useful in cases such as these—they decrease inflammation. I also would recommend multifidus-strengthening exercises in this case, as they would help to stabilize this person's spine, which we know it likely needs because it has severe aging changes. Recall that the normal course of these aging changes is that they bring about increased motion (remember the three phases of aging changes in the spine?). By helping control and decrease motion in the vertebrae with multifidus-strengthening exercises, you would be able to cut down on the irritation to the inflamed spinal nerve and foster recovery.

As you can see, surgery is not an absolute in a case like this. Unfortunately, when people have low-back pain and hear the phrases "severe degenerative changes" and "nerve compression" they have a tendency to lean toward surgical options to solve their back problems. Hopefully, now that you have a few more facts on hand about the spine and back pain, you can see that having "degenerative" changes in your back neither sentences you to surgery nor dooms you to a life of back pain.

Will a Back Belt Help My Back Pain?

The answer to this question isn't as straightforward as it may seem. Whether a back belt (also called back supports or lumbar corsets) will be beneficial for your back depends on why you're wearing it. Two scenarios pop into my mind:

- A person has no back pain at all and wears a support in hopes of *preventing* it.

- A person already has low-back pain and wears a back support to help them feel better and *treat* the pain.

As you can see, both people are wearing a back support, but for two totally different reasons. So the real questions are:

- Are back supports effective in preventing low-back pain?

and

- If you already have low-back pain, do back supports help decrease pain and improve function?

Nothing's ever as clear-cut as it seems, is it? To make matters worse, I recently read that there are over thirty types of lumbar supports made for the treatment of back disorders and more than seventy types for prevention. This all makes it very confusing for a person with back pain who just wants some relief! With all this in mind, I took a look at the literature with the previous questions in mind. Here's what I found:

Back Supports for Prevention

- The majority of studies deal with people who had non-specific low-back pain (no specific source of pain identified).

- ⊙ Studies were mainly done in occupational settings, on workers.

- ⊙ I found four studies that were randomized, controlled trials where one group got a back belt, and another group got nothing.

- ⊙ Not a single one of the studies showed any significant differences at follow-up between the two groups. It appears then, from the available literature, that you get the same amount of back pain regardless if you wear a back support or not.

Back Supports for Treatment

- ⊙ I was only able to locate one randomized, controlled trial that compared a group that wore a back support to a group that did not wear one (Penrose 1991).

- ⊙ It looked at patients with muscular sprain/strain of the low back. It did not specify the mean duration of the patient's complaints.

- ⊙ This study showed improved pain after one-hour, three-week, and six-week follow-ups in the group that wore the lumbar supports.

Based on the available evidence, I do not see any proof that back supports do actually prevent back pain. Four randomized, controlled trials have failed to show any significant differences between workers who wear them, and workers who don't. Incidentally, this is also the opinion of NIOSH, the National Institute of Occupational Safety and Health. They too find insufficient proof to support their use in preventing low-back pain.

On the other hand, we do have some evidence from a single randomized, controlled trial that shows a person with a simple "muscular strain" may benefit from wearing a back support. This study did have a short follow-up period though, so we don't really know what happened in the long run. Also, because the study failed to specify if these were acute or chronic low-back pain patients, I have no way of knowing which patient population benefits best from this treatment.

My *advice* is to try one if you like, but there are much better treatment options than lumbar supports to put your energy into.

If a Slipped Disk Is Pressing on a Nerve in My Back, Don't I Have to Have Surgery?

This is an area filled with many misconceptions and misunderstandings. I'm going to answer this one in several parts to try and give you a better overview of surgery and the slipped (or herniated) disk. First I'll address the question of whether the herniated disk pressing on a spinal nerve is really the cause of your pain.

- Sixty-four percent of people with *no* back pain can show a disk abnormality on an MRI test.

- Twenty-four percent of people with no back pain can show a compressed nerve on a myelogram test.

- A spinal nerve does not cause pain unless it is irritated and inflamed first.

- Not *all* pain going down the leg from the back is caused by a herniated disk. It has been demonstrated in studies that many structures in your back, when irritated, can send pain into the legs.

- Compressed nerves can cause neurological signs such as pain in certain patterns (called *dermatomes*) down the leg, or decrease one's strength, reflexes, and sensation in the lower extremities.

- These neurological signs should match and correlate well with any other additional diagnostic tests ordered, such as EMGs, MRIs, CT scans, and so on. However, relying just upon the results of these additional diagnostic tests in and of themselves to pinpoint the cause of the problem is a mistake without making sure that they really correspond with a person's symptoms.

Second, let's assume now that it has been determined that a herniated disk compressing a spinal nerve in your back is the true cause of your pain. One wonders at this point how surgery compares to conservative treatments (like traction, exercise, chiropractic, etc.) in the management of a problem like this. After all, why go through surgery if the problem can be managed with the same success or better without it? We return then to our old friend, the randomized, controlled trial. Here's what my literature search on this topic revealed:

- There is only one randomized, controlled trial that has compared surgery to conservative treatment in patients with lumbar disk herniations.

- This study was done by Henrik Weber and published in *Spine* in 1983.

- It looked at 126 patients with confirmed herniated lumbar disks with uncertain indications for surgery.

- One group got surgery, the other conservative therapy.

- Groups were followed at one, four, and ten years after treatment.

- At one year, the surgery group was doing better than the conservative group.

- At four- and ten-year follow-ups, there were no longer any significant differences between the surgery and conservative-therapy groups.

The conclusion from the available evidence? While the short-term results are better with surgical treatment for a herniated lumbar disk patient with uncertain surgical indications, it makes little difference in the long run whether you are treated conservatively or with surgery. One might then ask, if the results are ultimately the same, why not have surgery and feel better sooner? Well, there are some very undesirable changes that can occur from surgery, such as scar tissue formation around nerves and direct damage to the back muscles. I would recommend avoiding these serious changes if at all possible.

I'll begin the third part of this discussion by assuming that you have all the facts at hand and decide to go ahead and proceed with surgery. An informed consumer would of course want to know the success rate of surgery. One of the best studies I could locate was done by Loupasis in 1999. Here are a few details:

- The study followed 109 patients for seven to twenty years (average follow-up period was 12.2 years) who had undergone a standard diskectomy (surgical removal of a disk).

- Satisfactory results were found in 64 percent of patients studied.

- Twenty-eight percent still complained of significant back or leg pain.

- Seven point three percent of patients had a repeat operation.

- The authors concluded that the long-term results of standard disectomy were not very satisfying.

Maybe you're having second thoughts about surgery after taking in all this information. But on the other hand, your pain may be terrible, and there *is* a slipped disk pressing on a nerve. What will eventually happen to the disk if it isn't surgically removed? Does it just sit there, causing problems for the rest of your life? I wondered this myself some time ago and then did what I always do when I want to get to the bottom of things— conduct a literature search to find out what the research has uncovered. This is information I wish was passed around more often.

What eventually happens to a disk treated without surgery?

- Numerous studies have been done that have watched patients with confirmed herniated disks for varying periods of time.

- Most studies used a CT scan or MRI to follow the changes in the disk with the passage of time.

- Patients were all treated conservatively—that is, without surgery.

- All the studies I could locate revealed similar conclusions. *The majority of disk herniations can decrease in size substantially over a period of months without any type of surgical intervention.*

Mother Nature may indeed be the best healer of all. This is highly encouraging news for a person with a herniated-disk problem and has been well documented in many articles, to boot. It seems that if we basically leave well enough alone, the body has the potential to heal and improve itself.

So what role does the multifidus have in all of this? No, there are no randomized, controlled trials yet that have taken a group of people with documented herniated disks and put some of them in a control group and others in a treatment group that just did multifidus-strengthening exercises. This is what it would take to provide evidence that the treatment is really effective. So let me tell you what evidence we do currently have about using multifidus exercises with herniated-disk problems and you can decide for yourself if it's enough evidence to use them or not.

- ⊙ It has been documented that a herniated disk causes the multifidus muscle to be overactive and contract more than it should.

- ⊙ Samples taken of the multifidus muscle from patients undergoing surgery for disk herniations have shown the fibers to be much smaller than normal.

- ⊙ There have been studies done which have included back muscle exercises as part of a treatment program for herniated disk patients that have shown high rates of success. The problem here is that other treatments in addition to the strengthening exercises were also used, making it hard to say which particular treatment helped the most.

I think that strengthening the multifidus muscle has great potential to help treat patients with herniated-disk problems, although nothing conclusive can really be said yet about its effectiveness. We have so far identified problems with the multifidus muscle in patients with herniated disks, so it would make sense to try to correct those deficiencies with exercise. Strengthening the multifidus muscle will not directly treat the disk pressing on the nerve, but the exercises can correct the secondary problems the disk is causing (mentioned above). Also, as the research suggests, if the multifidus is not functioning properly, stability at that level of the spine is surely compromised. Getting the multifidus in shape with strengthening exercise can only help to regain stability at the level of the disk herniation. More stability means less irritation to the inflamed disk and nerve, creating an environment that fosters healing. I can only speculate that maybe this could even help the disk to decrease in size faster, since we know from follow-up studies that disks have a tendency to shrink over time. All we need now is a good randomized, controlled trial to see if multifidus-strengthening exercises can really get the job done.

What Are McKenzie Exercises?

The name "McKenzie exercises" means different things to different people, especially in the physical-therapy world. The name "McKenzie" refers to Robin McKenzie, a physical therapist known for his unique approach for treating back pain. McKenzie exercises typically refer to exercises where a person bends their spine backwards, either while standing or while lying on their stomach. An example is leaning backwards while standing. Backward bending of the spine is also known as *extension*, and so a lot of people refer to McKenzie exercises as "extension exercises."

This kind of stuff has irritated me to no end since I started my career as a physical therapist. Here's why. A long time ago, it was something called "Williams flexion exercises" that were in vogue. These exercises involve a patient bending their spine forward, usually while on their back. An example of this would be if you lay on your back and then bring both knees up to your chest. As you can see, this is the exact *opposite* motion of the McKenzie extension exercises. Lately I've been thinking about devising my own set of exercises for back pain that have one bend the spine *sideways* and call them, "Jim sidebending exercises." No wonder there's so much confusion when it comes to low-back pain!

While I definitely have a bone to pick with these types of therapies, I will try to be fair and stick to just the facts when discussing them. In *Physical Therapy of the Low Back*, McKenzie has said himself that his approach is often misunderstood. He wants to make it clear that his approach does not treat all patients with just extension exercises. Some he does treat with flexion (forward bending the spine) and even uses manipulation, if needed.

The McKenzie approach is really hard to characterize. An evaluation using the McKenzie approach monitors patient's responses to various back motions. McKenzie states that the success of his system depends on the "training and expertise of the physician and therapist especially." He also feels that "2 years of clinical experience with assessment and treatment of mechanical spinal disorder, coupled with appropriate education and certification, are minimum requirements for effective education in this method."

At this point, you may be asking yourself why McKenzie has chosen the extension (or backward bending) exercise as the mainstay of his treatment for many back problems. The reason has to do with the "centralization phenomenon" that is well documented in the research. If a person has pain that travels down into the legs, *centralization* is when it starts to work its way back up the leg until the pain has gradually "centralized" to just the low back. Pain that has centralized carries a better prognosis and usually subsides after centralizing. This can happen on its own, but has also been documented as happening when one bends the spine backward repeatedly. In all fairness, it should be restated again that while one could legitimately call this the heart of McKenzie's therapy, it's not the only treatment tool the McKenzie method uses in treating back patients. McKenzie also emphasizes other modalities such as posture, especially while sitting, and advocates the use of a lumbar roll to support the low-back curve for some patients.

Some of you may also be wondering why bending backward helps decrease back and leg pain. The thinking is that this backward bending motion of the spine causes the jelly-like center of the disk (the nucleus pulposus) to shift forward. This supposedly takes pressure off structures such as the spinal nerves or the back portion of the disk fibers, thereby relieving symptoms.

Upon conducting my own investigation of this most interesting method of treating low-back pain patients, I came across several problems.

- ⊙ The McKenzie method, at least the extension (backward bending) exercise portion, could probably not be used with patients who have spinal stenosis, spondylolisthesis, or problems with the facet joints.

- ⊙ Spinal stenosis patients have smaller than normal spinal canals and/or openings where the spinal nerves pass through, usually due to aging changes. Backward bending of the spine causes both of these spaces to narrow and become even smaller, further crowding out the spinal cord and nerves—not a good thing.

- ⊙ Patients with spondylolisthesis (slippage of one vertebra on the other, usually in a forward direction) can have cracks between the joints that allow the vertebrae to slip. Backward bending places more stress on this area, which can cause further slippage and make the problem worse.

- ⊙ The little joints of the spine (called the facet joints) are compressed and placed under more stress when one bends backward. A person with a facet-joint problem will likely not tolerate extension exercises.

◉ The McKenzie method has reliability problems. I was able to locate three studies that specifically examined reliability issues pertaining to this method.

◉ In basic terms, a McKenzie evaluation classifies patients as having one of three syndromes: a postural syndrome, a dysfunction syndrome, or a derangement syndrome. Kilby (1990) reported the level of agreement between therapists for each diagnosis. Therapists used an algorithm based on the McKenzie system. The percentage agreement for the dysfunction syndrome was 66.6 percent, the postural syndrome 100 percent, and the derangement syndrome 57 percent. It seems from these results that it's not easy to get therapists to agree on which syndrome a patient actually has.

◉ Riddle (1993) studied the intertester reliability of physical therapist's assessments of low-back pain patients using the McKenzie system. Reliability was found to be poor and therapists could only agree on which syndrome was present a disappointing 39 percent of the time, making this another study showing it to be difficult for two people using this system to decide exactly what a patient's problem really is.

◉ Donahue (1996) studied the intertester reliability of a modified version of McKenzie's lateral shift assessment using physical therapists evaluating low-back pain patients. According to McKenzie, the lateral shift is a lateral (sideways) displacement of a patient's trunk in relation to the pelvis. Evaluating for this shift is part of the McKenzie evaluation. The percentage agreement between the therapists was 47 percent, and the authors concluded that the role of the lateral shift assessment in the McKenzie system should be reconsidered.

But all that aside, does the McKenzie system really work? When the rubber meets the road, do patients actually improve? To try and answer these questions in an unbiased manner, we return once again to the results of the randomized, controlled trials. However, this is where it gets confusing. There were many studies that examined extension exercises in the treatment of low-back pain, but this is not really McKenzie therapy. I therefore excluded them, since extension exercises are just a part of McKenzie's program. I was then able to locate only three randomized, controlled trials that did use the McKenzie system. All of them looked at acute/subacute low-back pain, so this would mean that the patients in these studies all had pain less than three months in duration. Here's a brief review of the literature:

- ◉ Nwuga (1985) compared the McKenzie method to Williams flexion exercises and found that patients did better with the McKenzie treatment.

- ◉ Stankovic (1990, 1995) compared the McKenzie method to a mini back school in one study. Their follow-up study compared results at five years. Once again, patients in the McKenzie group fared better at both the one- and five-year follow-ups.

- ◉ Cherkin (1998) compared the McKenzie method, chiropractic manipulation, and an educational booklet. The authors found the McKenzie method and chiropractic manipulation to have similar effects and costs. However, both the McKenzie treatments and the chiropractic manipulation groups did only slightly better than those patients who simply received an educational booklet.

At first glance, it may seem as though all back-pain patients should be using the McKenzie method. I mean, for gosh sakes, two out of the three randomized, controlled trials showed the McKenzie system superior to the other comparison treatments.

But that's just the problem. What two of these good randomized, controlled trials have succeeded in proving is just that. The McKenzie method is superior to some treatments, but since none of the trials had a group of patients that received a placebo or no treatment at all, we still do no know whether the McKenzie approach can beat back pain's natural course of recovery. Remember that all these studies were done on acute and subacute back-pain patients. The prognosis for patients at this stage of low-back pain is actually quite good (see chapter 3). In other words, did the patients in the first two studies get better because of the McKenzie approach, or was it merely natural recovery? Only a control group of patients receiving no treatment at all compared to the McKenzie treatment could truly answer this question for us.

I don't recommend using McKenzie in the acute and sub-acute stages of low-back pain because there are much easier and cheaper alternatives to getting patients better than using an elaborate system that has published reliability problems. For instance, there are studies that show that the majority of patients with acute and subacute back pain can recover quite nicely with simple treatments such as analgesics and the advice to stay active while simply letting Mother Nature do the rest. Recall the results of the last trial above showing the McKenzie approach and chiropractic manipulation to be only *marginally* better than a simple educational booklet.

As for people with chronic low-back problems (back pain for longer than three months), which are probably the majority of readers, I am unable to locate any randomized, controlled trials at all that have used the McKenzie approach to treat this kind of back pain. Since there is no evidence one way or the other, the jury is still out on this one. Here again, my suggestion is to invest the time, energy, and money in other therapies that *have* demonstrated their effectiveness in multiple randomized, controlled trials, especially those therapies that have done better than another group that received minimal or no treatment at all.

Why Does My Back Pain Get Worse When I'm Under Stress?

My best guess is that your back muscles tighten up as a reaction to the stress, thereby making any existing back problem worse. However, the exact pathway that makes this happen is still a subject of much research.

As of yet, I have no conclusive proof that this is truly the case. However, avid readers of the clinical back literature, such as myself, are starting to see more and more literature each year dealing with the psychological influences on back pain.

In my *opinion*, there are at least two sides to back pain—the psychological side and the physical (or structural) side. These two sides are present and working to varying degrees in every case of back pain. The old structural paradigm that dominated in the past of back pain being caused by purely physical causes is now starting to fall apart. As an example, we now know that people can have herniated disks pressing on nerves and still walk around with no pain whatsoever. So what makes a herniated disk painful to some backs but not to others?

This is where the ever-increasing body of research on the psychological aspects of back pain is attempting to fill the gaps. Let me briefly share with you some of the most interesting research I have read about this topic to give you food for thought.

Bigos (1992) followed over three thousand employees at the Boeing-Everett Plant for four years to evaluate risk factors that might predispose workers to report back injuries. The researchers found job task dissatisfaction to be the individual factor that could best predict that an employee would report a back injury. It was not a physical factor such as back flexibility, strength, curve of spine, and so on.

Marras (2000) studied twenty-five people without back pain and looked at their trunk muscle activity and mechanical loading of their spine as they bent over and lifted boxes. Subjects performed the lifts under both stressed and unstressed conditions. Personality traits, blood pressure, and anxiety levels were assessed. Here are a few of their findings:

- The load on the back (such as compression) was more when subjects lifted boxes under stress than when they lifted under no stress.

- Certain personality types were linked to higher loads on the spine while lifting boxes. As an example, both introverts and intuitors had one of the biggest reactions to psychosocial stress, showing increases in lateral (side to side) shear and compression forces in the back while lifting under stress in comparison to the other personality types.

- When a box was lifted during a stressful situation, there was more back muscle activity noted than when a subject lifted in a nonstressful situation.

Linton (2000) conducted a review of the psychological risk factors involved in one getting back and neck pain. The problem with looking at risk factors such as depression predisposing or causing one to have back pain is that it can be hard to tell which came first. Did one have back pain and then become depressed, or was one depressed and then got the back pain? To get around this problem, Linton looked at mainly prospective studies. These are studies that collect information on people free of the problem being studied and then follow them over a period of time. At the end of the study, one then compares (as an example) those subjects that developed back pain to those who didn't. This helps one sort out cause and effect. The prospective study is the opposite of a *retrospective* study, where the researchers get information after the back pain has already developed. It is quite inferior to a prospective study because of such factors as observer bias and memory recall. Here are a few findings pertinent to our discussion from Linton's review:

- ◎ Thirty-seven studies of a prospective design, the best design for looking at the cause and development of a problem, were reviewed for the evidence regarding psychological factors in neck and back pain.

- ◎ Eleven studies were found that looked at anxiety, stress, and distress. All found a significant association between neck or back pain and these factors.

- ◎ Sixteen studies looked at mood and depression. Fourteen of them found that a depressed mood increases one's chances of getting a pain problem.

- ◎ Self-perceived poor health was found to be related to chronic pain and disability.

- ◎ Passive coping was associated with disability and pain.

- ◎ The prospective studies in Linton's review also showed that psychological factors are not only associated with the *onset* of back and neck pain, but are clearly linked to an acute problem turning into a chronic (long-term) problem.

Now you know why I said at the beginning of this section that the old structural paradigm of back pain being caused by purely physical causes is starting to fall apart. Good reviews such as the one above are shedding new light on low-back pain problems and alerting us to the fact that we must take *all* variables into account, both psychological and physical, if we really want to get people better.

By doing the multifidus-strengthening exercises in this book, you will be treating the physical component of your back pain. However, as the current literature suggests, other factors may also be involved. My suggestion is to consider some of the psychological factors above and see if they might be playing any kind of a role in your back problem, especially if you suffer from chronic back pain. By doing this, you cover all your bases, eliminating any factors that might be either precipitating or perpetuating your pain. Much scientific evidence is now starting to accumulate that backs up the mind-body connection, and this just might be an untapped area you can treat to finally eliminate this multidimensional problem.

7

Useful Information

I find that a great part of the information I have was acquired by looking up something and finding something else on the way.

—Franklin P. Adams

To me, it's of utmost importance that patients be as educated as possible about their low-back pain. I do not expect, however, that a patient will read, keep up with, and understand the scientific literature—that's the job of your medical professional.

So why have this chapter at all then? Well, for two good reasons. The first is that I feel compelled, for many reasons, to support what I write. If you have read any research or scientific literature, one of the first things you will notice are the little numbers at the end of some of the sentences, like this (1). These numbers, which match references at the end of the article, tell the reader where the author gets his information from.

I would like to have done this throughout this book; however, many publishers have told me that the general public does not like this and it makes the book read like a thesis. So, you can find the sources for the information I've provided on the references list if you wish, but you can also find information about other particular topics in this section.

The other reason to include a chapter such as this one is to provide useful information for readers if the need arises. Some people will read this book, do the exercises, and be quite happy at that. And that's okay. On the other hand, some might be curious about where the information comes from and will want to see the sources. A few readers will have questions about certain areas of the book and may even doubt the content and want to look it up for themselves. That's fine, too. In fact, I encourage it—you're a patient after my own heart. But whatever the case may be, this part is here for you to use as you see fit.

I've organized this section by topics. This should make it easier to find information on a particular subject that you might be interested in. If an article sparks your interest, and you desire to see the entire journal article, I suggest going to your nearest medical library, looking under the appropriate journal name (such as *Spine*) in the book stacks, finding the proper volume (the number after the journal name) and page numbers, and then simply photocopying it from there. If this all seems too daunting a task, I might add that I have yet to go to a medical library and not find extremely helpful staff members there waiting to help out.

In any event, try just browsing through the following list. I think at the very least, you'll find reading the titles of some of these articles very interesting and entertaining, as well as educational.

Anatomy of the Multifidus Muscle

Kalimo, H., J. Rantanen, T. Viljanen, et al. 1989. Lumbar muscles: Structure and function. *Annals of Medicine* 21:353–359.

What the Multifidus Muscle Does According to the EMG Studies

Arokoski, J. P. A., et al. 1999. Back and hip extensor muscle function during therapeutic exercises. *Archives of Physical Medicine and Rehabilitation* 80:842–850.

Donisch, E. W., and J. V. Basmajian. 1972. Electromyography of deep back muscles in man. *American Journal of Anatomy* 133:25–36.

Morris, J. M., G. Benner, and D. B. Lucas. 1962. An electromyographic study of the intrinsic muscles of the back in man. *Journal of Anatomy* 96:509–520.

Pauly, J. E. 1966. An electromyographic analysis of certain movements and exercises. I. Some deep muscles of the back. *Anatomical Record* 155:223–234.

Valencia, F. P., and R. R. Munro. 1985. An electromyographic study of the lumbar multifidus in man. *Electromyography and Clinical Neurophysiology* 25:205–221.

Structural Findings and Their Association with Low-Back Pain

Andersson, G. 1997. The epidemiology of spinal disorders. In *The Adult Spine*, vol. 1, 2nd ed., edited by J. W. Frymoyer. Philadelphia: Lippincott-Raven.

Imaging Tests and Abnormal Findings in People with No Back Pain

Hitselberger, W. E., and R. M. Witten. 1968. Abnormal myelograms in asymptomatic patients. *Journal of Neurosurgery* 28:204–206.

Jensen, M. C., et al. 1994. Magnetic resonance imaging of the lumbar spine in people without back pain. *New England Journal of Medicine* 331:69–73.

Wiesel, S. W., et al. 1984. A study of computer assisted tomography. I. The incidence of positive CAT scans in an asymptomatic group of patients. *Spine* 9:549–551.

Structural Abnormalities of the Multifidul Muscle Found in Only 1 to 5 Percent of Normal Subjects

Rantanen, J., A. Rissanen, and H. Kalimo. 1994. Lumbar muscle fiber size and type distribution in normal subjects. *European Spine Journal* 3:331–335.

Weber, B. R., et al. 1997. Posterior surgical approach to the lumbar spine and its effect on the multifidus muscle. *Spine* 22:1765–1772.

Changes in the Multifidus Muscle Found in Patients with Herniated Disks

Haig, A. J., et al. 1993. Prospective evidence for change in paraspinal muscle activity after herniated nucleus pulposus. *Spine* 18:926–930.

Mattila, M., et al. 1986. The multifidus muscle in patients with lumbar disk herniation. A histochemical and morphometric analysis of intraoperative biopsies. *Spine* 11:732–738.

Yoshihara, K., et al. 2001. Histochemical changes in the multifidus muscle in patients with lumbar intervertebral disk herniation. *Spine* 26:622–626.

Zhao, W., et al. 2000. Histochemistry and morphology of the multifidus muscle in lumbar disk herniation. Comparative study between diseased and normal sides. *Spine* 25:2191–2199.

Zhu, X., et al. 1989. Histochemistry and morphology of erector spinae muscle in lumbar disk herniation. *Spine* 14:391–397.

The Multifidus Muscle after Back Surgery

Kawaguchi, Y., H. Matsui, and H. Tsuji. 1996. Back muscle injury after posterior lumbar spine surgery. A histologic and enzymatic analysis. *Spine* 21:941–944.

Rantanen, J., et al. 1993. The lumbar multifidus muscle five years after surgery for a lumbar intervertebral disk herniation. *Spine* 18:568–574.

See, D. H., and G. H. Kraft. 1975. Electromyography in paraspinal muscles following surgery for root compression. *Archives of Physical Medicine and Rehabilitation* 56:80–83.

Changes in the Multifidus Muscle Found in Patients with Hypermobile Vertebrae

Lindgren, K. A., et al. 1993. Exercise therapy effects on functional radiographic findings and segmental electromyographic activity in lumbar spine instability. *Archives of Physical Medicine and Rehabilitation* 74:933–939.

Sihvonen, T., and J. Partanen. 1990. Segmental hypermobility in lumbar spine and entrapment of dorsal rami. *Electromyography and Clinical Neurophysiology* 30:175–180.

Changes in the Multifidus Muscle Found in Patients with Acute, Subacute, and Chronic Low-Back Pain

Hides, J. A., et al. 1996. Multifidus muscle recovery is not automatic after resolution of acute, first-episode low back pain. *Spine* 21:2763–2769.

Hides, J. A., M. J. Stokes, M. Saide, G. A. Jull, and D. H. Cooper. 1994. Evidence of lumbar multifidus muscle wasting ipsilateral to symptoms in patients with acute/subacute low back pain. *Spine* 19:165–172.

Parkkola, R., U. Rytokoski, and M. Kormano. 1993. Magnetic resonance imaging of the disks and trunk muscles in patients with chronic low back pain and healthy control subjects. *Spine* 18:830–836.

Strength-Training Principles

Feigenbaum, M. S., and M. L. Pollock. 1999. Prescription of resistance training for health and disease. *Medicine and Science in Sports and Exercise* 31:38–45.

The Sitting Posture

Adams, M. A., and W. C. Hutton. 1986. The effect of posture on the role of the apophyseal joints in resisting intervertebral compressive forces. *Journal of Bone and Joint Surgery* (Brit.) 62:358–362.

———. 1985. The effect of posture on diffusion into lumbar intervertebral disks. *Journal of Anatomy* 147:121–134.

———. 1985. The effect of posture on the lumbar spine. *Journal of Bone and Joint Surgery* 67-B:625–629.

Hedman, T. P., and G. R. Fernie. 1995. In vivo measurements of lumbar spinal creep in two seated postures using MRI. *Spine* 20:178–183.

Inufusa, A., et al. 1996. Anatomic changes of the spinal canal and intervertebral foramen associated with flexion-extension movement. *Spine* 21:2412–2420.

The Spine, the Disk, and Aging

Butler, D., et al. 1990. Disks degenerate before facets. *Spine* 15:111–113.

Kirkaldy-Willis, W. H., et al. 1978. Pathology and pathogenesis of lumbar spondylosis and stenosis. *Spine* 3:319–328.

Back Belts

Jellema, P., et al. 2001. Lumbar supports for prevention and treatment of low back pain. A systematic review within the framework of the Cochrane back review group. *Spine* 26:377–386.

What Happens to a Herniated Disk Treated without Surgery?

Bozzao, A., et al. 1992. Lumbar disk herniation: MR imaging assessment of natural history in patients treated without surgery. *Radiology* 1185:135–141.

Maigne, J. Y., et al. 1992. Computed tomographic follow-up study of 48 cases of non-operatively treated lumbar intervertebral disk herniation. *Spine* 17:1071–1074.

Saal, J. A., et al. 1990. The natural history of lumbar intervertebral disk extrusions treated non-operatively. *Spine* 15:683–686.

References

Bandy, W. D., and J. M. Irion. 1994. The effect of time on static stretch on the flexibility of the hamstring muscles. *Physical Therapy* 74:845–852.

Bandy, W. D., J. M. Irion, and M. Briggler. 1997. The effect of time and frequency of static stretching on flexibility of the hamstring muscles. *Physical Therapy* 77:1090–1096.

Bigos, S. J., et al. 1992. A longitudinal, prospective study of industrial back injury reporting. *Clinical Orthopedics and Related Research* 279:21–34.

Cherkin, D. C., et al. 1998. A comparison of physical therapy, chiropractic manipulation, and provision of an educational booklet for the treatment of patients with low back pain. *New England Journal of Medicine* 339:1021–1029.

Coste, J., et al. 1994. Clinical course and prognostic factors in acute low back pain: An inception cohort study in primary care practice. *British Medical Journal* 308:577–580.

Donahue, M. S., D. L. Riddle, and M. S. Sullivan. 1996. Intertester reliability of a modified version of McKenzie's lateral shift assessments obtained on patients with low back pain. *Physical Therapy* 76:706–726.

Fahrni, W. H., and G. E. Trueman. 1965. Comparative radiological study of the spines of a primitive population with North

Americans and Northern Europeans. *Journal of Bone and Joint Surgery* (Brit.) 47:552–555.

Gilbert, J. R., D. W. Taylor, A. Hildebrand, and C. Evans. 1985. Clinical trial of common treatments for low back pain in family practice. *British Medical Journal* 291:791–794.

Haig, A. J., D. B. LeBreck, and S. G. Powley. 1995. Paraspinal mapping. Quantified needle electromyography of the paraspinal muscles in persons without low back pain. *Spine* 20:715–721.

Hides, J. A., et al. 1996. Multifidus recovery is not automatic after resolution of acute, first episode low back pain. *Spine* 21:2763–2769.

———. 2001. Long-term effects of specific stabilizing exercises for first-episode low back pain. *Spine* 26:E243–248.

Kilby, J., M. Stignant, and A. Roberts. 1990. The reliability of back pain assessment by physiotherapists, using a "McKenzie algorithm." *Physiotherapy* 76:579–583.

Leboeuf-Yde, C. 2000. Body weight and low back pain. A systematic literature review of 56 journal articles reporting on 65 epidemiological studies. *Spine* 25:226–237.

Lindgren, K.A., et al. 1993. Exercise therapy effects on functional radiographic findings and segmental electromyographic activity in lumbar spine instability. *Archives of Physical Medicine and Rehabilitation* 74:933–939.

Linton, S. J. 2000. A review of psychological risk factors in back and neck pain. *Spine* 25:1148–1156.

Loupasis, G. A., et al. 1999. 7 to 20-year outcome of lumbar discectomy. *Spine* 24:2313–2317.

Marras, W. S., et al. 2000. The influence of psychological stress, gender, and personality on mechanical loading of the lumbar spine. *Spine* 25:3045–3054.

Nachemson, A., et al. 2000. *Neck and Back Pain: The Scientific Evidence of Causes, Diagnosis, and Treatment.* Philadelphia: Lippincott, Williams, and Wilkins.

Nwuga, G., and V. Nwuga. 1985. Relative therapeutic efficacy of the Williams and McKenzie protocols in back pain management. *Physiother Pract* 1:99–105.

O'Sullivan, P. B., et al. 19973. Evaluation of specific stabilizing exercise in the treatment of chronic low back pain with radiologic diagnosis of spondylolysis or spondylolisthesis. *Spine* 22:2959–2967.

Penrose, K. W., K. Chook, and J. L. Stump. 1991. Acute and chronic effects of pneumatic lumbar supports on muscular strength, flexibility, and functional impairment index. *Sports Train Med Rehabil* 2:121–129.

Riddle, D. L., and J. M. Rothstein. 1993. Intertester reliability of McKenzie's classifications of the syndrome types present in patients with low back pain. *Spine* 18:1333–1344.

Risch, S. V., et al. 1993. Lumbar strengthening in chronic low back pain patients. Physiologic and psychological benefits. *Spine* 18:232–238.

Rissanen, A., et al. 1995. Effects of intensive training on the isokinetic strength and structure of lumbar muscles in patients with chronic low back pain. *Spine* 20:333–340.

Roberts, G. M., et al. 1978. Lumbar spinal manipulation on trial, part II: Radiological assessment. *Rheumatology and Rehabilitation* 17:54–59.

Saal, J. A., and J. S. Saal. 1989. Nonoperative treatment of herniated lumbar intervertebral disc with radiculopathy. An outcome study. *Spine* 14:431–437.

Sihvonen, T., et al. 1998. Functional changes in back muscle activity correlate with pain intensity and prediction of low back pain during pregnancy. *Archives of Physical Medicine and Rehabilitation* 79:1210–1212.

Stankovic, R., and O. Johnell. 1990. Conservative treatment of acute low back pain. A prospective, randomized trial: McKenzie method of treatment versus patient education in "mini back school." *Spine* 15:120–123.

———. 1995. Conservative treatment of acute low back pain. A 5-year follow-up study of two methods of treatment. *Spine* 20:469–472.

Stein, J., E. Baker, and Z. M. Pine. 1993. Medial paraspinal electro-myography: Techniques of examination. *Archives of Physical Medicine and Rehabilitation* 74:497–500.

Tertti, M. O., et al. 1991. Low back pain and disc degeneration in children: A case control MR imaging study. *Radiology* 180:503–507.

Twomey, L., et al. 2000. *Physical Therapy of the Low Back*. Philadelphia: Churchill Livingstone.

Van Tulder, M. W., B. W. Koes, and L. M. Bouter. 1997. Conservative treatment of acute and chronic non-specific low back pain. *Spine* 22:2128–2156.

Waddell, G. 1998. *The Back Pain Revolution*. London: Churchill Livingstone.

Weber, H. 1983. Lumbar disc herniation. A controlled, prospective study with ten years of observation. *Spine* 8:131–140.

Some Other
New Harbinger Titles

The Cyclothymia Workbook, Item 383X, $18.95

The Matrix Repatterning Program for Pain Relief, Item 3910, $18.95

Transforming Stress, Item 397X, $10.95

Eating Mindfully, Item 3503, $13.95

Living with RSDS, Item 3554 $16.95

The Ten Hidden Barriers to Weight Loss, Item 3244 $11.95

The Sjogren's Syndrome Survival Guide, Item 3562 $15.95

Stop Feeling Tired, Item 3139 $14.95

Responsible Drinking, Item 2949 $18.95

The Mitral Valve Prolapse/Dysautonomia Survival Guide, Item 3031 $14.95

Stop Worrying Abour Your Health, Item 285X $14.95

The Vulvodynia Survival Guide, Item 2914 $15.95

The Multifidus Back Pain Solution, Item 2787 $12.95

Move Your Body, Tone Your Mood, Item 2752 $17.95

The Chronic Illness Workbook, Item 2647 $16.95

Coping with Crohn's Disease, Item 2655 $15.95

The Woman's Book of Sleep, Item 2493 $14.95

The Trigger Point Therapy Workbook, Item 2507 $19.95

Fibromyalgia and Chronic Myofascial Pain Syndrome, second edition, Item 2388 $19.95

Kill the Craving, Item 237X $18.95

Rosacea, Item 2248 $13.95

Thinking Pregnant, Item 2302 $13.95

Call **toll free, 1-800-748-6273,** or log on to our online bookstore at **www.newharbinger.com** to order. Have your Visa or Mastercard number ready. Or send a check for the titles you want to New Harbinger Publications, Inc., 5674 Shattuck Ave., Oakland, CA 94609. Include $4.50 for the first book and 75¢ for each additional book, to cover shipping and handling. (California residents please include appropriate sales tax.) Allow two to five weeks for delivery.

Prices subject to change without notice.